Trust Carol J. Buck and Elsevier
to take you through the levels of coding success

P9-ELG-957

Step 4:
Professional Resources

Step 3:
Certify

With the resources you need for every level of coding success, Carol J. Buck and Elsevier are with you every step of your coding career. From beginning to advanced, from the classroom to the workplace, from application to certification, the Step Series products are your guides to greater opportunities and successful career advancement.

Step 2:
Practice

Step 1:
Learn

Keep climbing with the most trusted names in medical coding.

Author and Educator
Carol J. Buck, MS, CPC, CCS-P

Lead Technical Collaborator
Jackie L. Grass, CPC

B-00

Step 1: Learn

" A journey of a thousand miles begins with a single step."

— Lao-tzu

Congratulations! You are embarking on an exciting and rewarding career, and you have taken a great first step. Coding is a career that gives you a chance to pursue excellence at a variety of levels, and we are happy that you have chosen to start with our *Step* line of products. As lifelong coders and educators, we are dedicated to giving you the tools you need to succeed. ***So, get out there and code!***

— Carol J. Buck,
MS, CPC, CCS-P

— Jackie L. Grass,
CPC

Track your progress!

See the checklist in the back of this book
to learn more about your next step toward coding success!

2016
STEP-BY-STEP
Medical Coding

Carol J. Buck
MS, CPC, CCS-P

WORKBOOK

2016
STEP-BY-STEP
Medical Coding

Carol J. Buck
MS, CPC, CCS-P

Jackie L. Grass
CPC

Former Program Director
Medical Secretary Programs
Northwest Technical College
East Grand Forks, Minnesota

Lead Technical Collaborator
Coder III/Reimbursement Specialist
Grand Forks, North Dakota

ELSEVIER

ELSEVIER

3251 Riverport Lane
St. Louis, Missouri 63043

WORKBOOK FOR STEP-BY-STEP MEDICAL CODING,   ISBN: 978-0-323-38921-1
2016 EDITION

Copyright © 2016 by Elsevier Inc.
Previous editions copyrighted 2015, 2014, 2013, 2012, 2011, 2010, 2009, 2008, 2007, 2006,
2005, 2004, 2002.

No part of this publication may be reproduced or transmitted in any form or by any means,
electronic or mechanical, including photocopying, recording, or any information storage
and retrieval system, without permission in writing from the publisher. Details on how to
seek permission, further information about the Publisher's permissions policies and our
arrangements with organizations such as the Copyright Clearance Center and the Copyright
Licensing Agency, can be found at our website: www.elsevier.com/permissions.

This book and the individual contributions contained in it are protected under copyright by
the Publisher (other than as may be noted herein).

NOTE: The *2016 ICD-10-CM* and *2016 ICD-10-PCS* were used in updating this text.

NOTE: *Current Procedural Terminology, 2016,* was used in updating this text.

Current Procedural Terminology (CPT) is copyright 2015 American Medical Association. All
Rights Reserved. No fee schedules, basic units, relative values, or related listings are included in
CPT. The AMA assumes no liability for the data contained herein. Applicable FARS/DFARS
restrictions apply to government use.

Although for mechanical reasons all pages of this publication are perforated, only those pages
imprinted with an Elsevier Inc. copyright notice are intended for removal.

┌───┐
│   **Notices**   │
│   │
│ Knowledge and best practice in this field are constantly changing. As new research and │
│ experience broaden our understanding, changes in research methods, professional practices, │
│ or medical treatment may become necessary.   │
│   Practitioners and researchers must always rely on their own experience and knowledge in │
│ evaluating and using any information, methods, compounds, or experiments described │
│ herein. In using such information or methods they should be mindful of their own safety │
│ and the safety of others, including parties for whom they have a professional responsibility. │
│   With respect to any drug or pharmaceutical products identified, readers are advised to │
│ check the most current information provided (i) on procedures featured or (ii) by the │
│ manufacturer of each product to be administered, to verify the recommended dose or │
│ formula, the method and duration of administration, and contraindications. It is the │
│ responsibility of practitioners, relying on their own experience and knowledge of their │
│ patients, to make diagnoses, to determine dosages and the best treatment for each │
│ individual patient, and to take all appropriate safety precautions.   │
│   To the fullest extent of the law, neither the Publisher nor the authors, contributors, or │
│ editors, assume any liability for any injury and/or damage to persons or property as a matter │
│ of products liability, negligence or otherwise, or from any use or operation of any methods, │
│ products, instructions, or ideas contained in the material herein.   │
└───┘

International Standard Book Number: 978-0-323-38921-1

Director, Private Sector Education & Professional/Reference: Jeanne R. Olson
Content Development Manager: Luke Held
Senior Content Development Specialist: Joshua S. Rapplean
Publishing Services Manager: Julie Eddy
Book Production Specialist: Celeste Clingan
Manager, Art & Design: Julia Dummitt

Printed in the United States of America

Last digit is the print number: 9 8 7 6 5 4 3 2 1

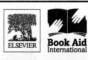

Working together
to grow libraries in
developing countries

www.elsevier.com • www.bookaid.org

Development of This Edition

QUERY MANAGER

Patricia Cordy Henricksen, MS, CHCA, CPC-I, CPC, CCP-P, ASC-PM
AAPC-Approved ICD-10-CM Trainer
Auditing, Coding, and Education Specialist
Soterion Medical Services/Merrick Management
Lexington, Kentucky

SENIOR COLLABORATOR AND ICD-10-CM CONSULTANT

Nancy Maguire, ACS, CRT, PCS, FCS, HCS-D, APC, AFC
Physician Consultant for Auditing and Education
Palm Bay, Florida

ICD-10-CM CONSULTANT

Kathy Buchda, CPC, CPMA
Revenue Recognition
Forest City, Iowa

EDITORIAL REVIEW BOARD

Brenda Parks Brown, HCA, MHS, CCS
Instructor
Roanoke, Virginia

Charlene A. Crump, CPC, AHI, CMAS
Financial Counselor
Healthspan
Cleveland, Ohio

Brenda J. Dombkowski, RMA, CPC, CPMA, CIMC
Compliance Auditor and Educator
New Haven, Connecticut

Mona F. Falcon, CPC, CMBS, CMAA, CCA
Academic Advisor
Laguna Hills, California

Pamela Harris-Brown, CMAS, CAHI, CPC, MBA
Coding Specialist/Coding Instructor
St. Louis, Missouri

Margaret Hengerle-Theodorakis, BS, RHIT, CPC, COC, CBCS
Instructor/Technical Writer
Virginia Beach, Virginia

Letitia Patterson, MPA, CPC, CCS-P
Consultant
A Coder's Resource
Chicago, Illinois

Rolando Russell, MBA/HCM, CPC, CPAR
Program Director/Healthcare Consultant
Ultimate Medical Academy
Tampa, Florida

Kathleen M. Skolnick, COC, CPC, CPCO, CPB, CPMA, CPPM, CPC-I, CEMC
Certified ICD-10-CM Instructor
Medical Coding for Professionals, LLC
Linden, New Jersey

Mary Lynn Taylor, MA-HIM, CMS, CPC, CPC-I
CEO
Professional Coding Services
Fairbanks, Alaska

LET THIS BE YOUR GOAL:

People who have accomplished worthwhile [goals] have had a very high sense of the way to do things. They have not been content with mediocrity. They have not confined themselves to the beaten tracks; they have never been satisfied to do things just as others do them, but always a little better. They always pushed things that came to their hands a little higher up, a little farther on. It is this little higher up, this little farther on, that counts in the quality of life's work. It is the constant effort to be first class in everything one attempts that conquers the heights of excellence.

Orison Swett Marden

This *Workbook* has been developed to assist you in the application of the theoretical and practical coding knowledge presented in the textbook *Step-by-Step Medical Coding*. The *Workbook* parallels the textbook with presentation of Chapters 1 through 27 and includes ample opportunity to practice the skill of medical coding. The *Workbook* contains three levels of questions—theory, abbreviated patient service and diagnosis descriptions, and original reports. The first level of question is the theory question; these questions are fill-in-the-blanks, multiple choice, true or false, and matching and often include medical terminology based on the specific area of coding presented in the coding manuals. The theory information serves as the foundational knowledge necessary to correctly code services and diagnoses. The second level of question is the abbreviated patient service and diagnosis descriptions; these questions begin the practical application of coding. The descriptions are condensed statements that provide broad-based coding experience. The final level is presented at the end of most *Workbook* chapters and contain reports that represent more complex services and diagnosis descriptions, such as operative, pathology, radiology, and emergency services.

The format for the answers has been developed to guide you in the development of your coding ability by using a format that includes four response variations:

- **One answer blank** for coding questions that require one code for the answer.
- **Multiple answer blanks** for coding questions that require more than one code for the answer.
- Key terms next to the blank(s) to guide you through the most difficult coding scenarios.
- **Answer blanks with ☜ preceding the blank to indicate that you must decide the number of codes necessary to correctly answer the question.**

Appendix B of the *Workbook* contains the answers to the odd-numbered questions, and the full answer key is available only in the TEACH Instructor Resources on Evolve. It is very important that you first complete the questions and then check your answers. The skill of medical coding can be acquired only through practice and by learning from mistakes that we all make along the way. It is from the understanding of why a service or diagnosis is coded in a certain way that you will develop a strong foundation that will serve you well throughout your coding career. Always take the time to read each code description fully, all notes connected with the code, and any applicable guidelines.

It is our sincere hope that you find the material presented in the *Workbook* challenging, enlightening, and worth your time and effort. Do your very best, and it will show in the quality of your work.

Carol J. Buck, MS, CPC, CCS-P
Jackie L. Grass, CPC

Some of the CPT code descriptions for physician services include physician extender services. Physician extenders, such as nurse practitioners, physician assistants, and nurse anesthetists, etc., provide medical services typically performed by a physician. Within this educational material the term "physician" may include "and other qualified health care professionals" depending on the code. Refer to the official CPT® code descriptions and guidelines to determine codes that are appropriate to report services provided by non-physician practitioners.

Contents

Some of the CPT code descriptions for physician services include physician extender services. Physician extenders, such as nurse practitioners, physician assistants, and nurse anesthetists, etc., provide medical services typically performed by a physician. Within this educational material the term "physician" may include "and other qualified health care professionals" depending on the code. Refer to the official CPT® code descriptions and guidelines to determine codes that are appropriate to report services provided by non-physician practitioners.

CHAPTER 1

Reimbursement, HIPAA, and Compliance

THEORY

Make sure to check **evolve** for the latest content updates

Without the use of reference material, answer the following:

1. What two groups of persons were added to those eligible for Medicare benefits after the initial establishment of the Medicare program?

   a. _____

   b. _____

2. To what government organization did the Secretary of the Department of Health and Human Services delegate the responsibility for administering the Medicare program?

   _____

3. What government organization handles the funds for the Medicare program?

   _____

4. There are three items that Medicare beneficiaries are responsible for paying before Medicare will begin to pay for services. What are these three items? _____, _____, and

   _____

5. Medicare publishes the Medicare fee schedule and usually pays what percentage of the amounts indicated for services? _____

6. The three components of work, overhead (practice expense), and malpractice are part of an RVU. What do the initials RVU stand for?

   _____

Odd-numbered answers are located in Appendix B, while the full answer key is only available in the TEACH Instructor Resources on Evolve.

Copyright © 2016 by Elsevier Inc.

7. According to the filing guidelines, providers must file claims for their

   Medicare patients within _____ months of the date of service.

8. What editions of the *Federal Register* would the outpatient facilities be
   interested in?

   _____ and _____

9. Under what act was a major change in Medicare in 1989 made possible?

   _____

10. Can a physician charge a patient to complete a Medicare form?

    _____

11. Individuals covered under Medicare are termed _____.

12. The _____ _____ _____
    do the paperwork for Medicare and are usually insurance companies
    that have bid for a contract with CMS to handle the Medicare program
    for a specific area.

13. Medicare Part C is also known as _____.

14. HIPAA stands for_____

    _____

15. The most major change to the health care industry as a result of HIPAA

    was as a result of what portion of the act? _____

    _____

16. The transfer of electronic documentation is accomplished through the

    use of _____ _____ Interchange technology.

17. The number that is assigned to all providers as a result of HIPAA:

    _____ _____ Identification

18. Under the Relative Value Unit system, _____ values are
    assigned to each service and are determined on the basis of the
    resources necessary to the physician's performance of the service.

19. The _____ charge historically was specific for each
    physician, but in 1993, the charge for a service was the same for all
    physicians within a locality, regardless of the specialty.

Odd-numbered answers are located in Appendix B, while the full answer key is only available in the TEACH Instructor Resources on Evolve.

Copyright © 2016 by Elsevier Inc.

20. For co-surgeons, Medicare pays the lesser of the actual charge or

    _____% of the global fee, dividing the payment equally between the two surgeons.

21. Specific regulations for Medicare are contained in the

    _____ _____ Manual.

22. Within an HMO, there is usually an individual who has been assigned to monitor the services provided to the patient both inside the facility and outside the facility. This person is known as the

    _____.

23. In this model of HMO, the HMO directly employs the physicians.

    _____ Model

24. In this model of HMO, the HMO contracts with the physician to provide the service at a set fee. These organizations are known as

    _____ _____ Associations.

25. An all-inclusive care program for the elderly that provides a comprehensive package of services that permits the client to continue

    to live at home is known as _____ for

    _____-_____ Care for the Elderly (PACE).

Odd-numbered answers are located in Appendix B, while the full answer key is only available in the TEACH Instructor Resources on Evolve.

CHAPTER 2

An Overview of ICD-10-CM

THEORY

Make sure to check
evolve
for the latest
content updates

Answer the following questions about the Overview of ICD-10-CM:

1. I-10 replaces I-9 Volumes 1 and 2.

   True   False

2. Mapping is a type of crosswalk to find corresponding diagnosis codes between I-9 and I-10.

   True   False

3. ICD-10 is widely used in Europe.

   True   False

4. The National Center for Health Statistics is responsible for the disease classification system in the United States.

   True   False

5. The 10th revision of the International Classification of Diseases (ICD-10) was issued in 1989 by the World Health Organization.

   True   False

6. The latest update for I-10 was in 2009.

   True   False

7. The I-10 contains 20 chapters.

   True   False

Odd-numbered answers are located in Appendix B, while the full answer key is only available in the TEACH Instructor Resources on Evolve.

8. All I-10 codes start with a letter and can have as many as 7 characters.

   True   False

9. GEMs refers to mapping files that crosswalk ICD-9-CM to ICD-10-CM and ICD-10-CM to ICD-9-CM.

   True   False

10. In the Tabular List, italicized type is used to identify codes not sequenced as first-listed diagnosis.

    True   False

11. Bold type is used throughout the entire Tabular List

    True   False

12. There are two tables located within the Index to Diseases and Injuries, hypertension and neoplasm.

    True   False

13. NOS (not otherwise specified) is equivalent of "unspecified."

    True   False

14. NEC is used when the I-10 code does not have codes that provide greater specificity.

    True   False

Identify the format of the chapters in the ICD-10-CM, Tabular List, in the proper sequence, from first to last:

15. _____   a. subcategory

16. _____   b. chapter

17. _____   c. subclassification

18. _____   d. section

19. _____   e. category

Odd-numbered answers are located in Appendix B, while the full answer key is only available in the TEACH Instructor Resources on Evolve.

Copyright © 2016 by Elsevier Inc.

PRACTICAL

Using the I-9 to I-10 GEMs file, map the following codes:

20. 401.9 _____   a. C50.919

21. V30.00 _____   b. R11.2

22. 787.01 _____   c. Y64.1

23. 174.9 _____   d. Z38.00

24. E875.1 _____   e. R10.12

25. 789.02 _____   f. I10

Using the I-10 to I-9 GEMs file, map the following codes:

26. A07.3 _____   a. 593.71

27. N13.721 _____   b. 719.84

28. Z98.810 _____   c. 250.60

29. M25.841 _____   d. 007.2

30. H81.8x9 _____   e. 386.8

31. E13.610 _____   f. V49.82

32. What does the Excludes1 note state under category C50?

_____

_____

33. What does the Includes note state under category I72?

_____

_____

34. Would code H36 be sequenced as the first-listed diagnosis?

_____

_____

Odd-numbered answers are located in Appendix B, while the full answer key is only available in the TEACH Instructor Resources on Evolve.

Copyright © 2016 by Elsevier Inc.

Using ICD-10-CM, Tabular List, locate the first pages of Chapter 9 and answer the following questions about the chapter:

35. The name of the chapter: _____

_____

36. The name of the first section: _____

_____

37. The description of the second category: _____

_____

38. The description of the first subcategory: _____

_____

39. What Excludes1 note applies to the first subcategory: _____

_____

Underline the main terms to be located in the Alphabetic Index in the following diagnostic statements:

40. Chronic pancreatitis

41. Anus abscess

42. Acute cholecystitis

43. Abdominal pain

44. Neonatal mastitis

Odd-numbered answers are located in Appendix B, while the full answer key is only available in the TEACH Instructor Resources on Evolve.

Copyright © 2016 by Elsevier Inc.

ICD-10-CM Outpatient Coding and Reporting Guidelines

THEORY

Using a current copy of the ICD-10-CM Guidelines for Coding and Reporting *for Outpatient Services, answer the following questions:*

1. Section IV Diagnostic Coding and Reporting Guidelines for Outpatient Services take precedence over the general and disease specific guidelines.

   True   False

2. Always begin the search for the correct code assignment in the Alphabetic Index.

   True   False

3. When a patient presents for outpatient surgery and the surgery is canceled, report the reason why the surgery was canceled as the first-listed diagnosis.

   True   False

4. The codes from A00 through Z99 are always reported as first-listed diagnoses.

   True   False

5. When a final diagnosis has not been established by the provider, it is acceptable to report codes for the presenting signs and symptoms.

   True   False

6. External Cause codes are located in the Alphabetical Index for Diseases under External Causes.

   True   False

Odd-numbered answers are located in Appendix B, while the full answer key is only available in the TEACH Instructor Resources on Evolve.

Copyright © 2016 by Elsevier Inc.

7. Report all conditions that coexist, even if they are not addressed or do not affect management/treatment during that encounter.

   True   False

8. For patients receiving diagnostic services only during an encounter/visit, sequence first the reason for the encounter/visit indicated in the medical record.

   True   False

9. A patient with primary lung cancer with metastasis to the spine presents for radiation treatment of the spine. The first-listed diagnosis reported is the primary lung cancer.

   True   False

10. For patients receiving preoperative evaluations, sequence first a code from the subcategory Z01.81, Encounter for preprocedural examinations, followed by findings related to the preoperative evaluation.

    True   False

11. Routine prenatal outpatient visits for high-risk patients are reported with a first-listed diagnosis from category O09, Supervision of high-risk pregnancy.

    True   False

12. Z codes may be reported as a principal diagnosis in the hospital setting.

    True   False

13. Heart transplant status code Z94.1 should not be reported with a code from subcategory T86.2, Complications of heart transplant.

    True   False

14. The External Cause codes can be reported as a first-listed diagnosis.

    True   False

15. When a patient is admitted to observation for a complication following outpatient surgery, report the complication as the first-listed diagnosis.

    True   False

Odd-numbered answers are located in Appendix B, while the full answer key is only available in the TEACH Instructor Resources on Evolve.

Copyright © 2016 by Elsevier Inc.

PRACTICAL

Assign ICD-10-CM first-listed diagnosis followed by additional diagnoses if appropriate:

16. Established 50-year-old patient with end-stage renal disease, currently receiving dialysis, is seen for acute left upper quadrant pain.

    First-listed Diagnosis: _____

    Code: _____

    Other Diagnosis: _____

    Code: _____

    Other Diagnosis: _____

    Code: _____

17. Established patient with complaints of shortness of breath. Upon examination, the physician determined she needed more aggressive treatment for her current congestive heart failure.

    First-listed Diagnosis: _____

    Code: _____

18. Patient is seen for unstable angina. He has a history of arteriosclerotic coronary artery disease.

    First-listed Diagnosis: _____

    Code: _____

19. Patient is seen for follow-up for hypertension. He has end-stage renal disease.

    First-listed Diagnosis: _____

    Code: _____

    Other Diagnosis: _____

    Code: _____

Odd-numbered answers are located in Appendix B, while the full answer key is only available in the TEACH Instructor Resources on Evolve.

20. Encounter for chemotherapy for prostate cancer.

    First-listed Diagnosis: _____

    Code: _____

    Other Diagnosis: _____

    Code: _____

21. Patient with chronic obstructive pulmonary disease (COPD) is seen for an acute lower respiratory tract infection.

    First-listed Diagnosis: _____

    Code: _____

22. Patient was scheduled for outpatient surgery for right inguinal hernia repair; however, he has a fever and a URI and the procedure is canceled.

    First-listed Diagnosis: _____

    Code: _____

    Other Diagnosis: _____

    Code: _____

    Other Diagnosis: _____

    Code: _____

23. An otherwise healthy patient is seen in the clinic for exposure to tuberculosis.

    First-listed Diagnosis: _____

    Code: _____

24. Patient presents for an outpatient chest x-ray, due to chest pain with breathing. Finding later indicated: normal x-ray.

    First-listed Diagnosis: _____

    Code: _____

Odd-numbered answers are located in Appendix B, while the full answer key is only available in the TEACH Instructor Resources on Evolve.

Copyright © 2016 by Elsevier Inc.

25. Patient, with known cardiovascular disease, is seen for a follow-up visit to discuss results of a cardiac perfusion study (cardiovascular function study), which was abnormal.

    First-listed Diagnosis: _____

    Code: _____

    Other Diagnosis: _____

    Code: _____

26. Following outpatient surgery for a right bunionectomy for hallux valgus, the patient was admitted to observation due to an exacerbation of her asthma post procedure.

    First-listed Diagnosis: _____

    Code: _____

    Other Diagnosis: _____

    Code: _____

27. A patient presents with a contusion to the left cheek that resulted from a fist fight, initial encounter.

    First-listed Diagnosis: _____

    Code: _____

    Other Diagnosis: _____

    Code: _____

28. Patient presents with a fracture of the right femur shaft due to a fall from her horse while riding, initial encounter.

    First-listed Diagnosis: _____

    Code: _____

    Other Diagnosis: _____

    Code: _____

    Other Diagnosis: _____

    Code: _____

Odd-numbered answers are located in Appendix B, while the full answer key is only available in the TEACH Instructor Resources on Evolve.

29. Encounter for insulin pump titration.

First-listed Diagnosis: _____

Code: _____

30. Patient in her second trimester is seen for a regular prenatal visit. She has a history of ectopic pregnancy.

First-listed Diagnosis: _____

Code: _____

31. Twin born via vaginal delivery, liveborn in the hospital.

First-listed Diagnosis: _____

Code: _____

32. Encounter for change of nephrostomy tube.

First-listed Diagnosis: _____

Code: _____

33. A patient was seen for an abrasion of the left upper arm, initial encounter.

First-listed Diagnosis: _____

Code: _____

34. Established patient is seen for hypertension and a prescription is refilled for psoriasis.

First-listed Diagnosis: _____

Code: _____

Other Diagnosis: _____

Code: _____

35. A patient who smokes 2 packs of cigarettes per day and suffers with chronic pulmonary disease is seen in follow-up for acute bronchitis.

First-listed Diagnosis: _____

Code: _____

Other Diagnoses: _____, _____

Code: _____, _____

Odd-numbered answers are located in Appendix B, while the full answer key is only available in the TEACH Instructor Resources on Evolve.

Copyright © 2016 by Elsevier Inc.

CHAPTER 4

Using ICD-10-CM

THEORY

Make sure to check evolve for the latest content updates

Without the use of reference material, answer the following:

1. An example of a late effect is hemorrhage after a surgery requiring a return to the operating room.

   True   False

2. You may report a code from the Index, without verifying in the Tabular when there is no indication that the code requires additional characters.

   True   False

3. If a patient has a confirmed diagnosis, the signs and symptoms related to that condition should also be reported.

   True   False

4. If the same condition is described as both acute and chronic, and separate subentries exist in the Alphabetic Index at the same indentation level, report both codes and sequence the acute code first.

   True   False

5. A dash (-) at the end of an Index entry indicates that an additional character or characters is/are required.

   True   False

6. Cholelithiasis with chronic cholecystitis without obstruction (K80.10) is an example of a dual code.

   True   False

7. A code is invalid if it has not been reported to the full number of characters available, including the 7th character, if applicable.

   True   False

Odd-numbered answers are located in Appendix B, while the full answer key is only available in the TEACH Instructor Resources on Evolve.

Copyright © 2016 by Elsevier Inc.

8. In most cases the manifestation codes will have in the code title, "in diseases classified elsewhere."

   True   False

9. A late effect usually occurs within 1 month of the illness or injury.

   True   False

10. In diabetic retinopathy, the retinopathy is the etiology and the diabetes is the manifestation.

    True   False

11. In the outpatient setting, it is correct to report a "probable" condition as if it exists, such as probable appendicitis as appendicitis.

    True   False

12. When sequencing codes for residuals and late effects, the late effect code is sequenced first followed by a code describing the residual condition.

    True   False

13. Section II of the *ICD-10-CM Official Guidelines for Coding and Reporting* includes instructions on outpatient coding and reporting.

    True   False

14. Diagnosis codes are always reported to the highest number of characters available.

    True   False

15. The cooperating parties for the development and approval of the *Official Guidelines for Coding and Reporting* are CMS, AMA, and NCHS.

    True   False

16. List two common symptoms associated with acute myocardial infarction.

    _____   _____

17. List two common symptoms associated with gastroesophageal reflux.

    _____   _____

18. List two common symptoms associated with seasonal allergies.

    _____   _____

Odd-numbered answers are located in Appendix B, while the full answer key is only available in the TEACH Instructor Resources on Evolve.

Copyright © 2016 by Elsevier Inc.

19. List two symptoms of a broken nose.

   _____ _____

Identify the Residual and Cause of the following diagnoses:

20. Acute renal failure due to previous viral encephalitis.

   Residual: _____

   Cause: _____

21. Constrictive pericarditis due to old tuberculosis infection.

   Residual: _____

   Cause: _____

22. Hemiplegia/hemiparesis affecting right dominant side due to cerebrovascular accident 4 months ago.

   Residual: _____

   Cause: _____

Odd-numbered answers are located in Appendix B, while the full answer key is only available in the TEACH Instructor Resources on Evolve.

Copyright © 2016 by Elsevier Inc.

PRACTICAL

Using the ICD-10-CM, code the following:

23. Acute and chronic sinusitis.

    ICD-10-CM Codes: _____, _____

24. Acute and chronic tonsillitis.

    ICD-10-CM Codes: _____, _____

25. Pneumoconiosis due to lime dust.

    ICD-10-CM Code: _____

26. Neuritis due to herniation of nucleus pulposus.

    ICD-10-CM Codes: _____, _____

27. Pneumonitis due to *Hemophilus influenzae.*

    ICD-10-CM Code: _____

28. Patient has unstable angina.

    ICD-10-CM Code: _____

29. Threatened shock, patient is hypotensive.

    ICD-10-CM Code: _____

30. Adult osteomalacia due to malnutrition.

    ICD-10-CM Code: _____

31. Pancreatitis, acute and chronic.

    ICD-10-CM Codes: _____, _____

32. Systemic lupus erythematosus causing endocarditis.

    ICD-10-CM Code: _____

33. Vitamin D-resistant rickets.

    ICD-10-CM Codes: _____, _____

34. Febrile complex convulsions with status epilepticus.

    ICD-10-CM Code: _____

35. Ascites in alcoholic hepatitis, alcohol use unspecified.

    ICD-10-CM Codes: _____, _____

Odd-numbered answers are located in Appendix B, while the full answer key is only available in the TEACH Instructor Resources on Evolve.

Copyright © 2016 by Elsevier Inc.

Chapter-Specific Guidelines (ICD-10-CM Chapters 1-10)

THEORY

Answer the following questions about the overview of ICD-10-CM:

1. Combination coding is when one code fully describes the conditions and/or manifestations.

   True   False

2. For hemiplegia and hemiparesis and other paralytic syndromes, report the right side as dominant if the documentation does not specify which side is dominant.

   True   False

3. When reporting an infection other than *Staphylococcus aureus*, that is antibiotic resistant, report the infection first followed by a code from category Z16, Infection with drug resistant microorganisms.

   True   False

4. Diabetes mellitus codes are combination codes that include the type of diabetes as well as the body system involved and complications affecting the body system.

   True   False

5. Methicillin-resistant *Streptococcus aureus* is also referred to as MRSA.

   True   False

6. For reporting purposes, urosepsis is not considered sepsis.

   True   False

7. If the medical documentation indicates the patient has two conditions that are both included in one diagnosis code, report that diagnosis code only once.

   True   False

Odd-numbered answers are located in Appendix B, while the full answer key is only available in the TEACH Instructor Resources on Evolve.

Copyright © 2016 by Elsevier Inc.

8. Multiple coding is when it takes more than one code to fully describe the condition, circumstance, or manifestation.

   True   False

9. When the histological type of neoplasm is documented, reference the Alphabetical Index first rather than going immediately to the Neoplasm Table.

   True   False

10. SIRS is the diagnosis when all of the following are diagnosed: hypothermia or fever, tachycardia, tachypnea, increased or decreased white blood count.

    True   False

11. Viral hepatitis codes are divided based on the type of hepatitis and if the condition is with or without hepatic coma.

    True   False

12. If a patient is admitted with pneumonia and while hospitalized develops severe sepsis, you would report the pneumonia first, followed by the severe sepsis.

    True   False

13. When an encounter is for treatment of anemia due to a malignancy, the first-listed diagnosis would be the malignancy, followed by the anemia.

    True   False

14. An "Uncertain" neoplasm is one that is not clearly benign or malignant.

    True   False

15. Septic shock is considered organ failure.

    True   False

16. Hepatitis A was formerly known as infectious or epidemic hepatitis.

    True   False

17. Epiphora is a blockage of the lacrimal passage.

    True   False

Odd-numbered answers are located in Appendix B, while the full answer key is only available in the TEACH Instructor Resources on Evolve.

Copyright © 2016 by Elsevier Inc.

18. When reporting hypertensive chronic kidney disease, an additional code to report the type of chronic kidney disease is not required.

    True   False

19. A Q-wave or transmural myocardial infarction, also known as STEMI, is the most severe type of infarction.

    True   False

20. Sepsis is classified as severe sepsis when it causes organ dysfunction.

    True   False

Odd-numbered answers are located in Appendix B, while the full answer key is only available in the TEACH Instructor Resources on Evolve.

PRACTICAL

Using the ICD-10-CM, code the following:

21. Acute renal failure and acute respiratory failure due to sepsis.

    ICD-10-CM Codes: _____, _____,

    _____, _____

22. A patient with early onset Alzheimer's progresses to combative behavior.

    ICD-10-CM Codes: _____, _____

23. Patient with known Hepatitis B seen in the clinic complaining of joint pain, loss of appetite, nausea and vomiting, and weakness and fatigue. He is admitted to the hospital for severe dehydration.

    ICD-10-CM Codes: _____, _____

24. An obstetric patient in her third trimester of pregnancy is admitted for *Pneumocystis carinii* pneumonia due to AIDS.

    ICD-10-CM Codes: _____, _____, _____

25. Lung abscess due to MRSA (Methicillin resistant *Staphylococcus aureus*).

    ICD-10-CM Codes: _____, _____, _____

26. Patient presents for HIV screening; patient is asymptomatic.

    ICD-10-CM Code: _____

27. Patient presents for follow-up exam following reconstructive surgery to repair hypospadias.

    ICD-10-CM Codes: _____, _____

28. Initial encounter for a 45-year-old woman receiving her first cycle of chemotherapy for pancreatic cancer is seen in the emergency room for severe nausea and vomiting due to the chemotherapy. She is admitted for dehydration.

    ICD-10-CM Codes: _____, _____, _____

29. Patient seen in an outpatient clinic with ascites due to disseminated malignant neoplasm.

    ICD-10-CM Codes: _____, _____

Odd-numbered answers are located in Appendix B, while the full answer key is only available in the TEACH Instructor Resources on Evolve.

Copyright © 2016 by Elsevier Inc.

30. Hypertensive heart disease, with congestive heart failure.

    ICD-10-CM Codes: _____, _____

31. Patient seen for cellulitis of left lower leg. He is a type 2 diabetic controlled with oral medications. The cellulitis has elevated his blood glucose and the physician elects to treat with sliding scale insulin regime.

    ICD-10-CM Codes: _____, _____

32. A 62-year-old man admitted to the hospital from the emergency room diagnosed with a transmural Q wave infarction. He has ASHD and had a pacemaker placed 5 years ago.

    ICD-10-CM Codes: _____, _____, _____

33. Patient seen in consult by a high-risk obstetrician. She is two months pregnant and was diagnosed with a malignant neoplasm of the left breast.

    ICD-10-CM Codes: _____, _____

34. Initial encounter for a patient with sepsis due to a blood transfusion. He has hemophilia.

    ICD-10-CM Codes: _____, _____, _____

35. Patient with anemia due to prostate cancer.

    ICD-10-CM Codes: _____, _____

36. Patient is admitted for chemotherapy for primary liver cancer.

    ICD-10-CM Codes: _____, _____

37. Patient admitted to hospital for bowel obstruction. This patient is also hypertensive with chronic kidney disease, stage 5.

    ICD-10-CM Codes: _____, _____, _____

38. Patient is following up at her oncologist's office for treatment options of metastatic cancer to right axillary lymph nodes. She has a history of right upper-outer quadrant breast cancer, still receiving treatment.

    ICD-10-CM Codes: _____, _____

39. Patient underwent a biopsy of the brain. The pathology report indicates secondary cancer from the primary site of the breast. The patient had a left mastectomy 5 years ago and currently receives no treatment for breast cancer.

    ICD-10-CM Codes: _____, _____, _____

Odd-numbered answers are located in Appendix B, while the full answer key is only available in the TEACH Instructor Resources on Evolve.

Copyright © 2016 by Elsevier Inc.

40. Patient underwent fulguration of malignant bladder tumors.

    ICD-10-CM Code: _____

41. Patient with polycythemia vera presented to an outpatient clinic for a phlebotomy.

    ICD-10-CM Code: _____

42. A 45-year-old man seen in the office is diagnosed with right carpal tunnel syndrome.

    ICD-10-CM Code: _____

43. Initial encounter for failure of insulin pump causing an overdose of insulin and hypoglycemic coma. The patient is a type 1 diabetic.

    ICD-10-CM Codes: _____, _____, _____

44. Patient diagnosed with dementia with Lewy bodies.

    ICD-10-CM Codes: _____, _____

45. Patient admitted to the hospital for resection of a malignant lung tumor from the right upper lobe.

    ICD-10-CM Code: _____

46. A man arrested for disorderly conduct is brought to the emergency room. He is a known alcoholic-dependent patient. Alcohol blood level indicates intoxication.

    ICD-10-CM Code: _____

47. Patient with chest pain is admitted to the hospital. He is diagnosed with acute Q wave myocardial infarction.

    ICD-10-CM Code: _____

48. Initial encounter for cardiac arrest due to cocaine dependence.

    ICD-10-CM Codes: _____, _____, _____

49. Schizophrenic with disorderly conduct noncompliance with his medications.

    ICD-10-CM Codes: _____, _____, _____

50. Delirium tremors due to withdrawal from cocaine dependence.

    ICD-10-CM Code: _____

Odd-numbered answers are located in Appendix B, while the full answer key is only available in the TEACH Instructor Resources on Evolve.

Copyright © 2016 by Elsevier Inc.

51. Meningitis caused by measles.

    ICD-10-CM Code: _____

52. Mononeuropathy of right lower limb due to diabetes, type 2.

    ICD-10-CM Code: _____

53. Polyneuropathy and arthritis due to syphilis.

    ICD-10-CM Codes: _____, _____

54. Streptococcal arthritis.

    ICD-10-CM Codes: _____, _____

55. Patient admitted with left hemiplegia and cerebral palsy for evaluation for possible Baclofen pump to treat spasticity.

    ICD-10-CM Code: _____

User to decide number of codes necessary to correctly answer the question.

56. Bilateral sensorineural deafness following bacterial meningitis.

    ICD-10-CM Code(s): _____

57. Ménière's disease.

    ICD-10-CM Code(s): _____

58. Right carotid stenosis causing a cerebral infarct.

    ICD-10-CM Code(s): _____

59. Acute pulmonary edema due to left heart failure. Patient now intubated and on a respirator.

    ICD-10-CM Code(s): _____

 User to decide number of codes necessary to correctly answer the question.

Odd-numbered answers are located in Appendix B, while the full answer key is only available in the TEACH Instructor Resources on Evolve.

Copyright © 2016 by Elsevier Inc.

REPORT

In Appendix A of this workbook you will find a section titled Reports, which contains original reports. Read the report indicated below and supply the appropriate ICD-10-CM codes on the following lines:

60. Report 7

    🌐 ICD-10-CM Code(s): _____

61. Report 9

    🌐 ICD-10-CM Code(s): _____

62. Report 19

    🌐 ICD-10-CM Code(s): _____

63. Report 20

    🌐 ICD-10-CM Code(s): _____

64. Report 34

    🌐 ICD-10-CM Code(s): _____

65. Report 39

    🌐 ICD-10-CM Code(s): _____

66. Report 40

    🌐 ICD-10-CM Code(s): _____

67. Report 42

    🌐 ICD-10-CM Code(s): _____

68. Report 44

    🌐 ICD-10-CM Code(s): _____

69. Report 90

    🌐 ICD-10-CM Code(s): _____

🌐 **User to decide number of codes necessary to correctly answer the question.**
Odd-numbered answers are located in Appendix B, while the full answer key is only available in the TEACH Instructor Resources on Evolve.

Copyright © 2016 by Elsevier Inc.

Chapter-Specific Guidelines (ICD-10-CM Chapters 11-14)

THEORY

Make sure to check
evolve
for the latest
content updates

Answer the following questions about the ICD-10-CM Guidelines for Coding and Reporting *for Outpatient Services:*

1. Includes and Excludes notes are only listed in the Tabular of the ICD-10-CM.

   True   False

2. Chapter 12, Diseases of the Skin and Subcutaneous Tissue, describes diseases or conditions of the integumentary and musculoskeletal systems.

   True   False

3. In the ICD-10-CM, pressure ulcers are graded and reported based on the depth of the ulcer.

   True   False

4. Code range M00-M02 reports infectious arthropathies due to infections that are direct or indirect.

   True   False

5. Chapter 13 of the *ICD-10-CM Guidelines for Coding and Reporting* indicates the 7th character D is assigned as long as the patient is receiving active treatment for a fracture.

   True   False

6. The two types of indirect infections are reactive and postinfective arthropathy.

   True   False

7. To report a hemorrhage, active bleeding must be present.

   True   False

Odd-numbered answers are located in Appendix B, while the full answer key is only available in the TEACH Instructor Resources on Evolve.

Copyright © 2016 by Elsevier Inc.

8. The categories in Chapter 11, Diseases of the Digestive System, begin when food enters the mouth and continue to when it leaves the body through the anus.

   True   False

9. Conditions affecting the nails, sweat glands, and hair are located in Chapter 12.

   True   False

10. The "Code first" note directs the coder to report first the underlying disease.

    True   False

Odd-numbered answers are located in Appendix B, while the full answer key is only available in the TEACH Instructor Resources on Evolve.

Copyright © 2016 by Elsevier Inc.

PRACTICAL

Using the ICD-10-CM, code the following:

11. Patient is seen for erosion of the teeth due to diet.

    ICD-10-CM Code: _____

12. Abscess of the salivary glands.

    ICD-10-CM Code: _____

13. Hemorrhage of the fallopian tube.

    ICD-10-CM Code: _____

14. Chronic prostatitis with hematuria.

    ICD-10-CM Codes: _____, _____

15. Cellulitis of female external genital organs.

    ICD-10-CM Code: _____

16. Stiffness of the right wrist.

    ICD-10-CM Code: _____

17. Congenital paraphimosis.

    ICD-10-CM Code: _____

18. Submandibular abscess.

    ICD-10-CM Code: _____

19. Secondary amenorrhea.

    ICD-10-CM Code: _____

20. Ligament disorder of the right foot joint.

    ICD-10-CM Code: _____

21. Patient suffers a nontraumatic hematoma of the soft tissue.

    ICD-10-CM Code: _____

22. Old sacroiliac joint lesion.

    ICD-10-CM Code: _____

Odd-numbered answers are located in Appendix B, while the full answer key is only available in the TEACH Instructor Resources on Evolve.

Copyright © 2016 by Elsevier Inc.

23. Inflammatory polyps of colon with intestinal obstruction.

    ICD-10-CM Code: _____

24. Hypertrophic scar.

    ICD-10-CM Code: _____

25. Chronic ulcer of the right thigh, non-pressure, with exposure of fat layer.

    ICD-10-CM Code: _____

26. Acute recurrent sialoadenitis.

    ICD-10-CM Code: _____

27. Unilateral internal inguinal hernia with gangrene, recurrent.

    ICD-10-CM Code: _____

28. Acute osteomyelitis of the right radius and ulna.

    ICD-10-CM Code: _____

29. Chronic nephritic syndrome with focal glomerulonephritis.

    ICD-10-CM Code: _____

30. Patient with end-stage renal disease, currently on hemodialysis.

    ICD-10-CM Codes: _____, _____

31. Infected pilonidal fistula with abscess.

    ICD-10-CM Code: _____

32. Cradle cap.

    ICD-10-CM Code: _____

33. Interstitial myositis of the left lower leg.

    ICD-10-CM Code: _____

34. Abnormal uterine bleeding, unrelated to menstrual cycle.

    ICD-10-CM Code: _____

35. Systemic lupus erythematosus with lung involvement.

    ICD-10-CM Code: _____

Odd-numbered answers are located in Appendix B, while the full answer key is only available in the TEACH Instructor Resources on Evolve.

Copyright © 2016 by Elsevier Inc.

36. *Staphylococcus aureus* arthritis of right carpal bones.

    ICD-10-CM Codes: _____, _____

37. Streptococcal group B arthritis of the metacarpus and phalanges, left hand.

    ICD-10-CM Codes: _____, _____

38. Endometriosis of the left ovary and fallopian tube.

    ICD-10-CM Codes: _____, _____

39. Patient is seen for a foreign body granuloma of the soft tissue, right upper arm.

    ICD-10-CM Code: _____

User to decide number of codes necessary to correctly answer the question.

40. Acute appendicitis with peritonitis with perforation of appendix.

    🔵 ICD-10-CM Code(s): _____

41. Chronic abscess of the areola of the right breast, unrelated to the puerperium.

    🔵 ICD-10-CM Code(s): _____

42. Cyst of the Bartholin's gland.

    🔵 ICD-10-CM Code(s): _____

🔵 **User to decide number of codes necessary to correctly answer the question.**
Odd-numbered answers are located in Appendix B, while the full answer key is only available in the TEACH Instructor Resources on Evolve.

Copyright © 2016 by Elsevier Inc.

31

REPORTS

In Appendix A of this workbook you will find a section titled Reports, which contains original reports. Read the reports indicated below and supply the appropriate ICD-10-CM codes on the following lines:

43. Report 6   ICD-10-CM Code(s): _____

44. Report 8   ICD-10-CM Code(s): _____

45. Report 10   ICD-10-CM Code(s): _____

46. Report 11   ICD-10-CM Code(s): _____

47. Report 12   ICD-10-CM Code(s): _____

48. Report 13   ICD-10-CM Code(s): _____

49. Report 14   ICD-10-CM Code(s): _____

50. Report 15   ICD-10-CM Code(s): _____

51. Report 31   ICD-10-CM Code(s): _____

52. Report 32   ICD-10-CM Code(s): _____

53. Report 33   ICD-10-CM Code(s): _____

54. Report 35   ICD-10-CM Code(s): _____

55. Report 38   ICD-10-CM Code(s): _____

56. Report 41   ICD-10-CM Code(s): _____

57. Report 43   ICD-10-CM Code(s): _____

58. Report 91   ICD-10-CM Code(s): _____

59. Report 92   ICD-10-CM Code(s): _____

60. Report 93   ICD-10-CM Code(s): _____

User to decide number of codes necessary to correctly answer the question.

Odd-numbered answers are located in Appendix B, while the full answer key is only available in the TEACH Instructor Resources on Evolve.

Copyright © 2016 by Elsevier Inc.

Chapter-Specific Guidelines (ICD-10-CM Chapters 15-21)

THEORY

Answer the following questions about the ICD-10-CM Guidelines for Coding and Reporting *for Outpatient Services:*

1. Chapter 17, Congenital Anomalies, can be reported any time during a person's life, as appropriate.

   True   False

2. Chapter 15 codes are never reported on the mother's record.

   True   False

3. The first-listed diagnosis for a routine outpatient prenatal visit is a code from category Z34, Encounter for supervision of normal pregnancy.

   True   False

4. The outcome of delivery is reported only on the newborn's record.

   True   False

5. The third trimester is considered 28 weeks 0 days from the first day of LMP until delivery occurs.

   True   False

6. A hydatidiform mole is a tumor that only forms in the uterus.

   True   False

7. When there is an encounter for a complication and no delivery occurred, report the complication as the first-listed condition.

   True   False

Odd-numbered answers are located in Appendix B, while the full answer key is only available in the TEACH Instructor Resources on Evolve.

Copyright © 2016 by Elsevier Inc.

8. When coding the birth episode in a newborn record, assign a code from Category Z38, Liveborn infants, according to place of birth and type of delivery, as the first-listed diagnosis.

    True   False

9. ICD-10-CM contains combination codes that identify only definitive diagnoses.

    True   False

10. The aftercare Z codes should not be reported for aftercare of injuries.

    True   False

11. Multiple fractures are sequenced in accordance to the location of the fracture.

    True   False

12. Corrosions are a result of a chemical contact and are classified by the depth, extent, and corrosive agent.

    True   False

13. You would assign an adverse effect code when a drug that was correctly prescribed and administered resulted in an adverse effect.

    True   False

14. When reporting multiple burns, sequence first the code that reports the highest degree of burn.

    True   False

15. Functional quadriplegia is the lack of ability to use one's limbs and is not associated with neurologic deficit or injury.

    True   False

With the use of reference material, answer the following:

16. When assigning one of the O10 codes that include hypertensive heart disease or hypertensive chronic kidney disease, it is necessary to add a

    _____ code from the appropriate hypertension category to specify the type of heart failure or chronic kidney disease.

17. A(n) _____ is an abnormality of a structure or organ.

Odd-numbered answers are located in Appendix B, while the full answer key is only available in the TEACH Instructor Resources on Evolve.

Copyright © 2016 by Elsevier Inc.

18. A _____ is defined as objective evidence of a disease that

    can be observed by the physician. A _____ is a subjective observation reported by the patient.

19. One method to locate abnormal findings in the Index of the I-10 is to

    reference the main term _____ and subterm by specific test.

20. Most categories in Chapter 19 of the ICD-10 have 7th character extensions. Most categories in this chapter have three extensions (with the exception of fractures): A, initial encounter, D, subsequent

    encounter, and _____, sequela.

21. A patient presents with second- and third-degree burns of the arm. What is the only degree of burn reported?

    _____

22. According to the guidelines on poisoning, _____ refers to taking less of a medication than is prescribed by a provider.

23. Codes from Chapter _____ of the Tabular of the I-10 report symptoms, signs, and abnormal clinical and laboratory findings.

24. Chapter _____ of the Tabular of the I-10 is probably the most difficult chapter from which to report diagnoses due to the complexity of coding.

25. According to the guidelines, when sequencing multiple fractures,

    sequence in accordance with the _____ of the fracture.

Odd-numbered answers are located in Appendix B, while the full answer key is only available in the TEACH Instructor Resources on Evolve.

Copyright © 2016 by Elsevier Inc.

PRACTICAL

Using the ICD-10-CM, code the following:

26. Induced abortion complicated by endometritis.

    ICD-10-CM Code: _____

27. Abrasion of the left upper arm, initial encounter.

    ICD-10-CM Code: _____

28. Hepatomegaly.

    ICD-10-CM Code: _____

29. Anaphylactic shock, initial encounter.

    ICD-10-CM Code: _____

30. Failure to gain weight, child.

    ICD-10-CM Code: _____

31. Pelvic peritonitis following ectopic pregnancy.

    ICD-10-CM Codes: _____, _____

32. Initial encounter of a patient transported to emergency department. Patient died from cardiac arrest due to an accidental overdose from heroin abuse.

    ICD-10-CM Codes: _____, _____, _____

33. Concealed penis.

    ICD-10-CM Code: _____

34. Crush syndrome, subsequent encounter.

    ICD-10-CM Code: _____

35. A 24-year-old woman at 32 weeks' gestation has hypotension.

    ICD-10-CM Code: _____

36. Newborn with cellulitis of the navel with mild hemorrhage.

    ICD-10-CM Code: _____

37. Inability to swallow.

    ICD-10-CM Code: _____

Odd-numbered answers are located in Appendix B, while the full answer key is only available in the TEACH Instructor Resources on Evolve.

Copyright © 2016 by Elsevier Inc.

38. Absence of bowel sounds.

   ICD-10-CM Code: _____

39. Sprain, left ankle, initial encounter.

   ICD-10-CM Code: _____

40. Newborn with obstructive sleep apnea.

   ICD-10-CM Code: _____

41. First- and second-degree burn, right hand, subsequent encounter.

   ICD-10-CM Code: _____

42. Partial traumatic amputation of the left index finger, initial encounter.

   ICD-10-CM Code: _____

43. Patient with persistent proteinuria.

   ICD-10-CM Code: _____

44. Accidental overdose of ibuprofen [NSAID], initial encounter.

   ICD-10-CM Code: _____

45. Hematoma of the nose, subsequent encounter.

   ICD-10-CM Code: _____

46. Newborn female delivered in the hospital by cesarean delivery.

   ICD-10-CM Code: _____

47. Fragile X syndrome.

   ICD-10-CM Code: _____

48. Anemia due to prematurity of infant.

   ICD-10-CM Code: _____

49. A 26-year-old woman at 30 weeks' gestation with quadruplets.

   ICD-10-CM Code: _____

Odd-numbered answers are located in Appendix B, while the full answer key is only available in the TEACH Instructor Resources on Evolve.

Copyright © 2016 by Elsevier Inc.

User to decide number of codes necessary to correctly answer the question.

50. Unexplained death, prior to entering health care facility.

    🔗 ICD-10-CM Code(s): _____

51. Tremors due to accidental overdose of monoamine oxidase, initial encounter.

    🔗 ICD-10-CM Code(s): _____

52. Nausea and vomiting.

    🔗 ICD-10-CM Code(s): _____

53. Blister of the right wrist, initial encounter.

    🔗 ICD-10-CM Code(s): _____

54. Acute gastritis with bleeding due to adverse effect of omeprazole, initial encounter.

    🔗 ICD-10-CM Code(s): _____

55. Subsequent encounter for fracture, right clavicle, with delayed healing.

    🔗 ICD-10-CM Code(s): _____

56. Positive occult blood in stools.

    🔗 ICD-10-CM Code(s): _____

57. Adult with respiratory distress and extreme fatigue.

    🔗 ICD-10-CM Code(s): _____

58. Vaginal pain.

    🔗 ICD-10-CM Code(s): _____

🔗 **User to decide number of codes necessary to correctly answer the question.**
Odd-numbered answers are located in Appendix B, while the full answer key is only available in the TEACH Instructor Resources on Evolve.

Copyright © 2016 by Elsevier Inc.

REPORTS

In Appendix A of this workbook you will find a section titled Reports, which contains original reports. Read the reports indicated below and supply the appropriate ICD-10-CM codes on the following lines:

59. Report 28

    🌐 ICD-10-CM Code(s): _____

60. Report 36

    🌐 ICD-10-CM Code(s): _____

61. Report 40

    🌐 ICD-10-CM Code(s): _____

62. Report 94

    🌐 ICD-10-CM Code(s): _____

63. Report 95

    🌐 ICD-10-CM Code(s): _____

🌐 **User to decide number of codes necessary to correctly answer the question.**
Odd-numbered answers are located in Appendix B, while the full answer key is only available in the TEACH Instructor Resources on Evolve.

Copyright © 2016 by Elsevier Inc.

8

Introduction to CPT

THEORY

Make sure to check
evolve
for the latest
content updates

Without the use of reference material, complete the following:

There were six index location methods presented in Chapter 8. List any four of the methods.

1. _____

2. _____

3. _____

4. _____

Match the appendix with the information it contains:

5. _____ Appendix E   a. Modifier -63 Information on Infants <4 kg

6. _____ Appendix F   b. Moderate Sedation

7. _____ Appendix G   c. Product Pending FDA Approval

8. _____ Appendix K   d. Modifier -51 exempt

9. You would expect to find the CPT code 71010 in what section of the CPT manual?

   _____

10. What is the report called that a physician dictates to show that an unusual or rare procedure is performed?

   _____

11. What association publishes the CPT?

   _____

Odd-numbered answers are located in Appendix B, while the full answer key is only available in the TEACH Instructor Resources on Evolve.

Copyright © 2016 by Elsevier Inc.

12. When you see the symbol ▲ in front of a code, you know what about the code?

_____

13. What type of code has the full code description? _____

14. What type of code has only a portion of the code description?

_____

15. What would providers enter on the insurance form to show payers which services or procedures were performed?

_____ and/or _____

16. The use of a coding system allows you to communicate not only

quickly, but also _____.

17. The first edition of the CPT was published in what year? _____

18. The updated CPT manual is available for purchase in what month?

_____

19. A standard for communicating health care data, as represented in CPT, was necessary to address requirements of this 1996 act:

_____

_____ and _____ Act.

20. What does the symbol of a circle with a line through it (⊘) placed before a CPT code indicate about the code?

_____

PRACTICAL

With the use of the CPT manual section Guidelines, identify the following unlisted codes:

Radiology

21. Clinical brachytherapy _____

22. Therapeutic radiology clinical treatment planning _____

23. Therapeutic radiology treatment management _____

Odd-numbered answers are located in Appendix B, while the full answer key is only available in the TEACH Instructor Resources on Evolve.

Copyright © 2016 by Elsevier Inc.

Pathology and Laboratory

24. Surgical pathology procedure _____

25. Urinalysis procedure _____

Medicine

26. Allergy/clinical immunological service _____

27. Special dermatological service _____

28. Dialysis procedures, inpatient or outpatient _____

Odd-numbered answers are located in Appendix B, while the full answer key is only available in the TEACH Instructor Resources on Evolve.

CHAPTER 9

Introduction to the Level II National Codes (HCPCS)

THEORY

Without the use of reference material, complete the following:

HCPCS is a collection of codes that may be provided to Medicare and Medicaid beneficiaries to represent these four items.

1. _____

2. _____

3. _____

4. _____

5. Level II codes (National Codes) are approved and maintained by this

   workgroup. _____

6. Level II National Modifiers are located in the introduction section of the

   HCPCS and also in what Appendix of CPT? _____

7. G codes are used to identify what type of procedures and services that would otherwise be reported with a CPT code but no CPT code has been established?

   _____

8. Medicare and other federal payers do not recognize "S" codes; however, "S" codes may be useful for claims to what type of insurers?

   _____

   List the temporary national codes letter for items or services reuniform national coding between one year's update and the next.

Copyright © 2016 by Elsevier Inc.

9. _____

10. _____

11. _____

12. HCPCS codes J9000-J9999 cover the cost of the chemotherapy drug. What is not included in payment for the reported J code?

_____

13. Items billed before a signed and dated order has been received by the supplier must be submitted with this modifier.

_____

14. This HCPCS modifier indicates a required Waiver of Liability was issued to the patient.

_____

15. HCPCS codes that are used to identify services that would not be reported with a CPT code, such as drugs, biologicals, and types of medical equipment/services, which are not identified by Level II National codes.

_____

Match the following administration methods for drugs:

16. _____ OTH   a. Subcutaneous

17. _____ IT   b. Inhalant solution

18. _____ IV   c. Various routes

19. _____ IM   d. Intrathecal

20. _____ SC   e. Intramuscular

21. _____ INH   f. Intravenous

22. _____ VAR   g. Other routes

Odd-numbered answers are located in Appendix B, while the full answer key is only available in the TEACH Instructor Resources on Evolve.

Copyright © 2016 by Elsevier Inc.

PRACTICAL

With the use of the HCPCS Level II manual section Guidelines, identify the following codes:

23. Abatacept _____

24. Bacterial sensitivity study _____

25. Carbon filter _____

26. Cerumen, removal _____

27. Ear mold, not disposable _____

28. Paclitaxel, 1 mg _____

29. Tire, wheelchair _____

30. Vaccine administration, influenza _____

31. Vaccine administration, pneumococcal _____

32. Walking boot, non-pneumatic, customized _____

Odd-numbered answers are located in Appendix B, while the full answer key is only available in the TEACH Instructor Resources on Evolve.

CHAPTER 10

Modifiers

THEORY

Without the use of reference material, answer the following:

1. What appendix in the CPT manual contains a complete list of all modifiers?

   _____

2. What is the word that means assigning multiple codes when one code would do?

   _____

3. What is the term that describes the services provided to a patient by the physician before surgery?

   _____

4. What is another term for the time after the surgery that the physician provides services to the patient?

   _____

5. Do all third-party payers recognize all modifiers as listed in the CPT manual?

   _____

6. What is the term that describes two physicians working together in the completion of a procedure when each has the same level of responsibility?

   _____

Odd-numbered answers are located in Appendix B, while the full answer key is only available in the TEACH Instructor Resources on Evolve.

Copyright © 2016 by Elsevier Inc.

PRACTICAL

Using the CPT and ICD-10-CM/ICD-9-CM manuals, indicate the modifiers and diagnoses that would be reported for the following:

7. A patient is admitted and has bilateral arthroscopy of the knees due to Baker's cysts.

   Modifier: _____

   ICD-10-CM Codes: _____ , _____

   (ICD-9-CM Code: _____)

8. Ben Carter, surgical resident, assists Dr. Wells, chief cardiologist, in a coronary artery bypass procedure due to coronary arteriosclerosis of a native artery. What modifier would be submitted to report Ben's services in the teaching hospital?

   Modifier: _____

   ICD-10-CM Code: _____

   (ICD-9-CM Code: _____)

9. Dr. Wells began surgery for right knee replacement due to severe osteoarthritis on an 86-year-old female with controlled hypertension. The patient was satisfactorily anesthetized and the site opened to view. Shortly thereafter, the patient's blood pressure dropped significantly, and the physician was unable to stabilize the patient. The procedure was discontinued.

   Modifier: _____

   ICD-10-CM Codes: _____ , _____

   (ICD-9-CM Codes: _____ , _____)

10. The patient is a 10-month-old boy who fell while trying to walk across the kitchen floor at his home. He suffered an open wound to his bottom lip. Sutures are necessary but due to the patient's age and excessive movement general anesthesia is needed.

    Modifier: _____

    ICD-10-CM Codes: Diagnosis: _____

    External Cause W Code: _____

    External Cause Y Code Place of Occurrence: _____

    (ICD-9-CM Codes: Diagnosis: _____)

Odd-numbered answers are located in Appendix B, while the full answer key is only available in the TEACH Instructor Resources on Evolve.

Copyright © 2016 by Elsevier Inc.

E Code Cause: _____

(E Code Place of Occurrence: _____)

11. A radiological examination of the gastrointestinal tract was ordered by a third-party payer for a confirmation of Crohn's disease (regional enteritis) of the large bowel. Crohn's was confirmed.

    Modifier: _____

    ICD-10-CM Code: _____

    (ICD-9-CM Code: _____)

12. Anesthesia provided by the ENT physician during a tympanoplasty for repair of a tympanic membrane perforation.

    Modifier: _____

    ICD-10-CM Code: _____

    (ICD-9-CM Code: _____)

13. A patient is seen at the direction of Workers' Compensation for a complete physical examination for insurance certification.

    Modifier: _____

    ICD-10-CM Code: _____

    (ICD-9-CM Code: _____)

14. The patient returns to the operating room by same physician for removal of deep pins during the postoperative period, due to complication (dislodged) after an open repair of a humerus fracture.

    Modifier: _____

15. A patient has a surgical procedure on Tuesday, and later that day the physician must take the patient back to the operating room to repeat (redo) a coronary bypass, due to complications of initial procedure.

    Modifier: _____

16. The patient underwent a bilateral tympanoplasty.

    Modifier: _____

17. If you must use two or more modifiers to describe a service, you would use which modifier to indicate this circumstance?

    Modifier: _____

Odd-numbered answers are located in Appendix B, while the full answer key is only available in the TEACH Instructor Resources on Evolve.

Copyright © 2016 by Elsevier Inc.

18. A surgeon performs a procedure on a neonate weighing 9 kg; the procedure was extremely complicated. What modifier would you use to indicate this service, which has an increased level of complexity?

    Modifier: _____

19. Dr. Storely performed cataract surgery on 10/31/20XX and Dr. Jones provided postoperative care following discharge. What modifier would you use to indicate the postoperative care following discharge?

    Modifier: _____

20. Dr. Merideth serves as an assistant surgeon to Dr. Taylor. What modifier would you add to the procedure code to indicate Dr. Merideth's status during the procedure?

    Modifier: _____

21. The third-party payer requires the use of HCPCS/National modifiers; the surgeon performed a surgical procedure on the patient's left thumb. What Level II modifier would indicate the left thumb?

    Modifier: _____

22. What Level II modifier indicates the upper left eyelid?

    Modifier: _____

Odd-numbered answers are located in Appendix B, while the full answer key is only available in the TEACH Instructor Resources on Evolve.

52

Copyright © 2016 by Elsevier Inc.

Evaluation and Management (E/M) Services

THEORY

Make sure to check **evolve** **for the latest content updates**

Without the use of reference material, complete the following:

1. _____ Consultation

2. _____ Admission

3. _____ Office visit

4. _____ Newborn care

5. _____ Established patient

6. _____ Inpatient

7. _____ New patient

8. _____ Outpatient

a. A face-to-face encounter in an office between the physician and patient

b. One who has not received professional service from the physician or another physician in the exact same specialty and subspecialty in the same group within the last 3 years

c. Advice or opinion from one physician to another physician

d. One who has been formally admitted to an acute health care facility

e. One who has received professional service from the physician or another physician in the exact same specialty and subspecialty in the same group within the last 3 years

f. Attention to an acute illness or injury that results in hospitalization

g. Evaluation and determination of care for a newborn infant

h. One who has not been formally admitted to a health care facility

Odd-numbered answers are located in Appendix B, while the full answer key is only available in the TEACH Instructor Resources on Evolve.

Copyright © 2016 by Elsevier Inc.

CHAPTER 11 ▪ Evaluation and Management (E/M) Services

The four types of medical decision making, in order of complexity from most to least complex, are as follows:

9. _____

10. _____

11. _____

12. _____

13. Complexity of medical decision making is based on three

_____.

List the five types of presenting problems from the most risk and least recovery to least risk and most recovery:

14. _____

15. _____

16. _____

17. _____

18. _____

19. Counseling and coordination of care are what kind of factors in most

cases? _____

20. Time that is used as a guide for outpatient services is what kind of time?

_____

Inpatient time spent at the bedside or nursing station during or after

the visit is what kind of time? _____

21. The patient's _____ _____ will reflect the number of systems examined by a brief statement of the findings.

22. A discussion with a patient and/or family concerning one or more of the following areas: diagnostic results, impressions and/or recommended diagnostic studies; prognosis; risks and benefits of treatment; instructions for treatment; importance of compliance with treatment; risk factor reduction; and patient and family education is

_____.

23. The history is the _____ information the patient tells the physician.

Odd-numbered answers are located in Appendix B, while the full answer key is only available in the TEACH Instructor Resources on Evolve.

Copyright © 2016 by Elsevier Inc.

24. There is no distinction made between the new and established patients

    in this service department of a hospital: _____

25. Those services rendered by a physician whose opinion or advice is
    requested by another physician or agency in the evaluation and/or

    treatment of a patient is a(n) _____, whereas the
    physician who has primary responsibility for the patient in the hospital

    is called _____.

26. When critically ill patients in medical emergencies require the constant
    attendance of the physician (e.g., cardiac arrest, shock, bleeding, and
    respiratory failure) to stabilize them, what kind of care is needed?

    _____

27. When care is provided for similar services (e.g., hospital visits) to the
    same patient by more than one physician on the same day for different

    conditions, the care is _____.

28. What is the name for the assumption of the total or specific care of a
    patient from one physician to another that does not constitute a

    consultation? _____

29. An inventory of body systems obtained through questioning to identify
    signs and/or symptoms that the patient may be experiencing is a(n)

    _____ of _____.

30. If the physician who is standing by does so for 25 minutes, can he or
    she round the time up to 30 minutes for reporting purposes?

    _____

**Odd-numbered answers are located in Appendix B, while the full answer key is only available in the TEACH
Instructor Resources on Evolve.**

PRACTICAL

Office or Other Outpatient Services and Hospital Inpatient Service

With the use of the CPT and ICD-10-CM/ICD-9-CM manuals, complete the following:

31. Analyze this case in which the patient record states: 40-year-old male patient (new) is evaluated for contusion of a finger. The history and examination were problem focused.

    a. Diagnosis and management options for contusion of finger. (Options can be minimal, limited, multiple, or extensive.) Diagnosis and

       management options: _____

       Data to review to provide service. (Data can be minimal/none, limited, moderate, or extensive.) Only data available are current

       information obtained during the visit. Data: _____

    b. Risks if left untreated. (Risk can be minimal, low, moderate, or high.)

       Risks: _____

    c. All three of the elements have been met to qualify this patient for

       what level of decision making complexity? _____

       _____

    d. The patient record indicates that a problem focused history and examination were done. When this is combined with the level of decision-making complexity you arrived at for this patient, what is

       the correct CPT code for the case? Code: _____

32. A patient who was on observation status for 48 hours is discharged from the hospital. The patient was being observed after a motor vehicle accident for subdural hematoma, subsequently ruled out. Code only the discharge services and diagnosis.

    CPT Code: _____

    ICD-10-CM Codes: _____, _____

    (ICD-9-CM Codes: _____, _____)

33. Initial observation of a patient was for upper abdominal pain, dizziness, and anemia. A comprehensive history and examination was performed. Moderate complexity decision making was conducted to admit the patient to observation to treat and rule out causes of the patient's anemia.

    CPT Code: _____

Odd-numbered answers are located in Appendix B, while the full answer key is only available in the TEACH Instructor Resources on Evolve.

Copyright © 2016 by Elsevier Inc.

34. A 16-year-old female is being admitted by her family practice physician with a 2-week history of fatigue and fever. It has been progressively getting worse. She is suffering from dehydration. The physician performs a comprehensive history to look for explanations for her fatigue, including recent activity level and recent sleep habits. A detailed examination is performed and she is diagnosed with mononucleosis and admitted for treatment.

    CPT Code: _____

    ICD-10-CM Codes: _____, _____

    (ICD-9-CM Codes: _____, _____)

35. A 56-year-old male with an established history of ASHD of native arteries and past stent placement is admitted through the emergency room with acute onset of chest pain. An EKG was performed and troponin levels taken. Both showed evidence of the patient having an acute inferior wall myocardial infarction. The cardiologist performs a comprehensive history, with the chief complaint, 4 from the history of present illness (HPI), a complete review of systems (ROS), and past, family, and social history (PFSH). The history includes the information that the pain started a week ago but last night worsened. Also on a scale of 1 to 10, he rated the pain an 8. It was also discovered that the patient has not been attending regular appointments in the clinic setting. A comprehensive examination was performed along with high-complexity medical decision making (MDM), including management of the patient's acute MI and reviewing data of the medical history of the patient. He was taken immediately to the cardiac catheterization lab to look for the source for the patient's MI.

    CPT Code: _____

    ICD-10-CM Codes: _____, _____, _____

    (ICD-9-CM Codes: _____, _____,

    _____)

36. The patient is a 34-year-old established patient seen in the clinic by her dermatologist. She is followed for extensive psoriasis involving her scalp, trunk, and arms. It has now worsened and spread to her palms, and she is now also complaining of joint pain. The spread to her hands has made it difficult to do many of her day-to-day tasks. A detailed history and examination are performed. The examination includes inspection of the affected areas in addition to bending and rotation of joints. A long discussion took place regarding a change in her medications to try to gain better control of her psoriasis and slow down the systemic progression. Topical and systemic treatment was decided on.

    CPT Code: _____

    ICD-10-CM Codes: _____, _____

    (ICD-9-CM Codes: _____, _____)

Odd-numbered answers are located in Appendix B, while the full answer key is only available in the TEACH Instructor Resources on Evolve.

Copyright © 2016 by Elsevier Inc.

37. A 2-year-old boy with bacterial pneumonia is hospitalized and has had 5 days of antibiotic therapy. Today the child developed a fever of 101° F with a mild rash on his torso. In a subsequent hospital visit, the attending physician performed a problem focused history and examination. The MDM complexity was low.

    CPT Code: _____

    ICD-10-CM Code: _____

    (ICD-9-CM Code: _____)

38. The patient is a 52-year-old male from out of state visiting his daughter. He left his medications for his benign hypertension at home and is now here in the clinic in need of a prescription. A problem focused history and examination is performed and a prescription is given to the patient.

    CPT Code: _____

    ICD-10-CM Code: _____

    (ICD-9-CM Code: _____)

Consultation Services

39. A 47-year-old female was sent by her family practice physician for an office consultation with a gynecologist. The patient has been suffering with moderate pelvic pain, a heavy sensation in her lower pelvis, and marked discomfort during sexual intercourse. In a detailed history, the gynecologist noted the location, severity, and duration of her pelvic pain and related symptoms. In the review of systems, the patient had positive findings related to her gastrointestinal, genitourinary, and endocrine body systems. The physician noted that her medical history was noncontributory to the present problem. The detailed physical examination centered on her gastrointestinal and genitourinary systems, with a complete pelvic examination. The physician ordered laboratory tests and a pelvic ultrasound to determine uterine fibroids, endometritis, or other internal gynecological pathology. The MDM complexity was moderate.

    CPT Code: _____

    ICD-10-CM Codes: _____, _____

    (ICD-9-CM Codes: _____, _____)

40. A 38-year-old female has severe low back pain due to a trauma injury she experienced as a factory worker 4 years ago. The chronic pain has become almost unbearable, and her internal medicine physician cannot go any further with her treatment. An initial outpatient consultation is requested and the patient is sent to see the pain management specialist for suggestions to control the chronic pain. A comprehensive history is taken, including all of the pertinent information regarding her injury. During the comprehensive examination the patient's gait and

Copyright © 2016 by Elsevier Inc.

movement were observed. Moderate-complexity decision making is performed, including different treatment options. A separate note is dictated to show the requesting physician what results were found during the visit and the decision on treatment of her pain.

CPT Code: _____

ICD-10-CM Codes: _____, _____

(ICD-9-CM Codes: _____, _____)

41. An inpatient urological consultation is performed for a 32-year-old female who recently had an elective abortion performed on an outpatient basis. The woman has been admitted with a high fever, pelvic pain, and dysuria. During a detailed history, the urologist notes in the history of present illness that the patient's symptoms began about 2 days after the abortion and progressed to the acute phase, which she is in at the present time. The location of the pain is in the lower abdomen and rated 9 on a scale of 1 to 10. She reports the quality of the pain to be sharp and stabbing. In the review of systems, the physician notes positive responses in 5 of the 12 body systems investigated. The urologist notes a negative medical history related to urinary symptoms other than a mild cystitis about 10 years ago. The detailed physical examination performed by the urologist centers on the genitourinary system and gastrointestinal system in significant detail. The medical decision making is low. Given the patient's past surgical procedure and physical findings at the present, the consultant considers the diagnoses of pyelonephritis, cystitis, pyelitis, and endometritis.

CPT Code: _____

42. A 46-year-old male is admitted to the hospital with a progressive staphylococcal pneumonia that is not responding to treatment. A request is made for the infectious disease physician on staff to render his opinion for treatment. The patient is seen in initial inpatient consultation. An expanded problem focused history and examination are performed. After looking at the sputum cultures, the physician decides on the most effective antibiotic for treatment. The decision making is straightforward.

CPT Code: _____

ICD-10-CM Code: _____

(ICD-9-CM Code: _____)

43. The initial consulting physician subsequently sees a 55-year-old patient injured at work when he fell from a house roof and struck his head. The patient had a right frontal parietal craniotomy 6 days previously and is recovering rapidly. The initial consultation was requested regarding a possible drug reaction that produced a rash on the upper torso. The consultant recommended a medication change, but after 48 hours the patient had no improvement. The physician re-evaluates for other possible causes of the rash. An expanded problem focused interval

Copyright © 2016 by Elsevier Inc.

history and a physical examination were performed. The MDM complexity was moderate.

CPT Code: _____

ICD-10-CM Code: _____

(ICD-9-CM Code: _____)

44. A 44-year-old patient, with chronic mastoiditis, was seen in consultation by the ENT specialist in the office. Her physician was inquiring as to the advantages of surgery versus continued antibiotic treatment when an acute flare comes on. The ENT specialist recommends surgery because of the increasing severity with each acute flare. She is fearful of the surgery because of the need to go under general anesthetic and a fear of permanent hearing loss. The physician performs an expanded problem focused history to include the duration of this problem and how many acute flares a year the patient experiences. An expanded problem focused examination and straightforward decision making is completed. It is determined that with the number of acute flares a year and the increasing severity of each case that surgery is recommended. The patient's fears are laid to rest and the patient decides to go ahead with the surgery.

CPT Code: _____

ICD-10-CM Code: _____

(ICD-9-CM Code: _____)

45. This is a follow-up visit on a 28-year-old male who is admitted with the diagnosis of headaches. The patient is subsequently seen because the physician needs to follow up on test results that weren't back yet at the initial consultation. This will help to find a possible cause of the headaches and course of treatment. A problem focused history and examination and low-complexity decision making is made after viewing the CT results. The diagnosis of tension headaches was made and treatment options discussed.

CPT Code: _____

ICD-10-CM Code: _____

(ICD-9-CM Code: _____)

46. An 83-year-old patient is seen at the local nursing home. The patient suffers from severe COPD. Routine labs were drawn on the patient by her primary doctor and her blood sugar came back abnormal. Fasting glucose was then taken and was high. The endocrinologist was asked to render an opinion on a possible diagnosis of diabetes. A problem focused history and examination and straightforward decision making were made. Diabetes was diagnosed and treatment started. The endocrinologist contacted the primary physician and discussed treatment of the patient. Report services for the endocrinologist only.

Odd-numbered answers are located in Appendix B, while the full answer key is only available in the TEACH Instructor Resources on Evolve.

Copyright © 2016 by Elsevier Inc.

CPT Code: _____

ICD-10-CM Code: _____

(ICD-9-CM Code: _____)

47. A patient is sent to a general surgeon by her family physician for an opinion and recommendation for surgical repair of a recurrent femoral hernia, right. A brief problem focused history of present illness and a problem focused examination of the affected body area and organ system are performed in the office. The MDM complexity was straightforward.

CPT Code: _____

ICD-10-CM Code: _____

(ICD-9-CM Code: _____)

48. A pulmonologist is asked, by the patient's primary physician, to see a 14-month-old boy who was admitted to the hospital with respiratory distress, cough, and fever. A comprehensive history is taken from the parents because this is an infant. It was determined that the patient does attend a day care facility. The cough and fever have been present for approximately 5 days. The infant started having trouble breathing this morning. The patient is intubated. Pneumonia due to respiratory syncytial virus is the definitive diagnosis. A comprehensive examination is performed along with moderate decision making. More tests will follow. A copy of his dictation will be sent to the primary physician.

CPT Code: _____

ICD-10-CM Code: _____

(ICD-9-CM Code: _____)

49. Office neurosurgery consultation is requested by the primary physician for a 32-year-old man on workers' compensation who is unable to work because of displacement of intervertebral lumbar disc with myelopathy. Two previous surgical repairs have been unsuccessful in relieving the patient's pain. The patient has been unable to return to his employment as a bricklayer. He complains of radiating pain throughout the buttocks and leg, with numbness throughout the leg and foot. Reflexes are minimal to nonexistent. A comprehensive history and physical examination are performed. MDM complexity was high due to the prior surgeries and continued complaints.

CPT Code: _____

ICD-10-CM Code: _____

(ICD-9-CM Code: _____)

Odd-numbered answers are located in Appendix B, while the full answer key is only available in the TEACH Instructor Resources on Evolve.

Emergency Department Services, Nursing Facility, Domiciliary, and Home Services

50. A patient presents to the emergency department after being involved in a motor vehicle accident. The patient was wearing a seat belt. The vehicle rolled numerous times. The patient's head struck the side window. The patient is unresponsive and is intubated. A history was unable to be obtained because of the patient's unresponsiveness. What history is available comes from the paramedics and patient's record. A comprehensive examination reveals the abdomen to be quite swollen with extensive bruising around the lower abdomen caused by the seat belt. High-complexity decision making was involved and the patient was rushed to the operating room.

    CPT Code: _____

51. A male patient presents to the emergency department with a wrist sprain sustained in a softball game when the patient slid into home, striking his hand on home plate. The patient is in apparent pain with a swollen wrist, which he is unable to flex. An expanded problem focused history and physical examination are done. Radiographs show a Colles' fracture of the distal radius. The MDM complexity was low.

    CPT Code: _____

    ICD-10-CM Codes: _____, _____, _____

    (ICD-9-CM Codes: _____, _____,

    _____)

52. An 88-year-old female's family physician comes to the nursing facility to perform the resident's annual assessment. A detailed interval history is taken with some information from the patient, but because of her limited cognitive abilities, most of the information is gathered from the nurses and past records. A comprehensive multisystem physical examination is performed, which includes extensive body areas and related organ systems. The MDM complexity was moderate because multiple diagnoses must be considered for this patient, who has senile dementia, diabetes, hypertension, hypothyroidism, and recurrent transient ischemic attacks. The creation of a new treatment plan is required because some of the patient's conditions have worsened.

    CPT Code: _____

    ICD-10-CM Codes: _____, _____,

    _____, _____, _____

    (ICD-9-CM Codes: _____, _____,

    _____, _____, _____)

Odd-numbered answers are located in Appendix B, while the full answer key is only available in the TEACH Instructor Resources on Evolve.

Copyright © 2016 by Elsevier Inc.

53. This is a home visit on an elderly gentleman, previously unknown to me, who is complaining of edema in his lower extremities. Pain is associated with this. An expanded problem focused history and examination are performed and low complexity decision making. Jobst stockings are prescribed.

    CPT Code: _____

    ICD-10-CM Code: _____

    (ICD-9-CM Code: _____)

54. Subsequent follow-up care is provided for the 82-year-old male nursing facility patient with Alzheimer's disease. The resident has responded well to some new medications and appears to have recovered some of his cognitive abilities without behavioral disturbances. The physician performs a problem focused history and physical examination on his neurological problem and orders the current treatments continued. The MDM complexity is low.

    CPT Code: _____

    ICD-10-CM Codes: _____, _____

    (ICD-9-CM Codes: _____, _____)

55. Subsequent follow-up care is provided for the patient who was transferred to a skilled nursing facility from an acute care hospital after partial recovery from a stroke. The patient has developed periods of extreme dizziness and mental confusion. A detailed interval history is gathered, and a detailed physical examination of the affected body systems is performed. Given the possibility that a new stroke could have occurred or that other neurological problems have developed, new orders are written, and the physician plans to return the next day to evaluate the patient's condition again. The MDM complexity is moderate.

    CPT Code: _____

    ICD-10-CM Codes: _____, _____, _____

    (ICD-9-CM Codes: _____, _____,

    _____)

56. The physician provides services to a resident of a rest home for an ulcerative sore on the heel and midfoot. Given the fact that the patient is in reasonably good health and is not diabetic, the physician focuses his attention on the right lower extremity during the problem focused physical examination. The physician knows the resident well and performs a brief HPI and ROS during a problem focused history. The resident thinks the sore is from new shoes, and the physician agrees

Odd-numbered answers are located in Appendix B, while the full answer key is only available in the TEACH Instructor Resources on Evolve.

Copyright © 2016 by Elsevier Inc.

63

with that conclusion. Topical antibiotic cream is ordered, and the new shoes are sent to the cobbler to be stretched. The MDM complexity is straightforward.

CPT Code: _____

ICD-10-CM Code: _____

(ICD-9-CM Code: _____)

57. The physician provides services to a new patient who is in a custodial care center. The patient is 43 years old and is paraplegic, with severe infected stasis ulcers. The physician performs a detailed history and examination and prescribes an antibiotic. The MDM was straightforward.

CPT Code: _____

Prolonged Services and Preventive Medicine Services

58. An established patient is seen in the office for a new problem that requires a comprehensive history and examination. The MDM complexity is high, and the physician spends 40 minutes with the patient. However, the patient has numerous concerns, and the physician spends an additional hour and 50 minutes in prolonged direct patient contact.

CPT Codes: _____, _____,

_____

59. A 44-year-old asthmatic patient (new) is scheduled for a routine office visit for a complaint of severe headaches. The physician provides a comprehensive history and examination. The MDM complexity was high. Toward the end of the visit, the patient develops severe breathing complications, and the physician spends the next hour and 30 minutes administering treatment.

CPT Codes: _____, _____,

_____

60. A 64-year-old man arrives at his appointment with his family physician for his annual physical examination. The patient has no new complaints and all of his medications remain the same. He is told to follow up in 1 year or sooner if necessary.

CPT Code: _____

Services from Throughout the E/M Section

61. A new patient is seen in the office for a variety of medical problems. The patient has insulin-dependent diabetes mellitus with complicating eye and renal problems. She also has hypertensive heart disease with episodes of congestive heart failure. Her peripheral vascular disease has

Odd-numbered answers are located in Appendix B, while the full answer key is only available in the TEACH Instructor Resources on Evolve.

Copyright © 2016 by Elsevier Inc.

worsened, and she can walk only a block before she is crippled with extreme leg pain. The patient reports that a new problem has surfaced: throbbing headaches with radiating neck pain. To manage and investigate the multiplicity of problems, the physician performs a comprehensive history and physical examination. A complete review of systems is performed, as is an update to her complete past, family, and social history. The physician has to take a multitude of factors into consideration because this patient's problems are highly complex.

CPT Code: _____

62. A new patient is seen in the office complaining of a sore throat and reports a low-grade fever for the past 4 days. The physician performs an expanded problem focused history and an expanded problem focused examination of the respiratory and lymphatic system. The physician's impression was acute pharyngitis and straightforward decision making was performed. Amoxicillin was prescribed.

CPT Code: _____

ICD-10-CM Code: _____

(ICD-9-CM Code: _____)

63. This is a 32-year-old female patient admitted for observation after an allergic reaction to her pain medication. She is alert and oriented, but has severe pruritus and shortness of breath. A detailed history and examination is performed after she takes medication for the pruritus; the breathing improved and the patient was discharged from observation on the same day.

CPT Code: _____

ICD-10-CM Codes: _____, _____,

_____

(ICD-9-CM Codes: _____, _____,

_____)

64. The patient was admitted to the hospital 3 days ago with severe dehydration and hyponatremia. The patient is now being discharged. Discharge takes 30 minutes.

CPT Code: _____

ICD-10-CM Codes: _____, _____

(ICD-9-CM Codes: _____, _____)

Odd-numbered answers are located in Appendix B, while the full answer key is only available in the TEACH Instructor Resources on Evolve.

Copyright © 2016 by Elsevier Inc.

65. A family practice physician who is treating a 20-year-old man (inpatient) for bronchitis calls in a urologist to examine the patient, who has requested a circumcision. The consultant performs a problem focused history and problem focused physical examination and determines that there is no urgency for the surgical procedure. The physician's decision making is fairly straightforward, and he recommends that the patient have the procedure done as an outpatient at a later date.

CPT Code: _____

66. A physician visits a 75-year-old female in the extended nursing facility as part of her annual assessment. The physician completes a detailed interval history with a comprehensive, head-to-toe physical examination. The physician reviews and affirms the medical plan of care developed by the multidisciplinary care team at the nursing facility. The patient's condition is stable; her hypertension and diabetes (type 2) are in good control and she has no new problems. The physician has limited data to review and few diagnoses to consider. The MDM complexity was low.

CPT Code: _____

ICD-10-CM Codes: _____, _____

(ICD-9-CM Codes: _____, _____)

67. A 67-year-old female is admitted with severe exacerbation of her COPD. The patient is now in respiratory failure and CHF. The patient is intubated and unconscious; 155 minutes of critical care time was spent at bedside and coordinating care for this patient.

⊛ CPT Code(s): _____

⊛ ICD-10-CM Code(s): _____

(⊛ ICD-9-CM Code(s): _____)

68. Henry Green, an established patient, came into the office for his yearly physical examination. Henry is 72 and in good health.

CPT Code: _____

ICD-10-CM Code: _____

(ICD-9-CM Code: _____)

⊛ User to decide number of codes necessary to correctly answer the question.

Odd-numbered answers are located in Appendix B, while the full answer key is only available in the TEACH Instructor Resources on Evolve.

Copyright © 2016 by Elsevier Inc.

REPORTS

In Appendix A of this workbook you will find a section titled Reports, which contains original reports. Read the reports indicated below and supply the appropriate CPT and ICD-10-CM/ICD-9-CM codes on the following lines:

69. Report 1

   CPT Code: _____

   ICD-10-CM Codes: _____, _____,

   _____

   (ICD-9-CM Codes: _____, _____,

   _____)

70. Report 2

   CPT Code: _____

   ICD-10-CM Codes: _____(secondary neoplasm),

   _____ (primary neoplasm), _____ (vena

   cava syndrome), _____ (catheter complication),

   _____ (hypertension), _____ (nerve pain),

   _____ (anemia, in (due to) (with), neoplastic disease)

   (ICD-9-CM Codes: _____, _____,

   _____, _____, _____,

   _____)

71. Report 3

   CPT Code: _____

   ICD-10-CM Code: _____

   (ICD-9-CM Code: _____)

72. Report 4

   CPT Code: _____

73. Report 5

   CPT Code: _____

Odd-numbered answers are located in Appendix B, while the full answer key is only available in the TEACH Instructor Resources on Evolve.

CHAPTER 12

Anesthesia

THEORY

Make sure to check evolve for the latest content updates

Without the use of reference material, answer the following:

1. What two words describe a decreased level of consciousness that does not put patients completely to sleep and that allows the patients to

   breathe on their own during a surgical procedure? _____

   _____

2. What do the initials CRNA stand for?

   _____

3. CMS publishes an annual list of _____ values for anesthesia codes.

4. The "M" in the anesthesia formula stands for _____ unit.

5. What is the term that describes the services provided to a patient by the physician before surgery?

   _____

6. What is another term for the time after the surgery when the physician provides services to the patient?

   _____

7. The _____ factor for the locale is multiplied by the number of base units in the procedure plus the time units to determine the price of the anesthesia service.

8. This modifier indicates that a CRNA service with medical direction by a physician was provided. _____

Odd-numbered answers are located in Appendix B, while the full answer key is only available in the TEACH Instructor Resources on Evolve.

Copyright © 2016 by Elsevier Inc.

PRACTICAL

With the use of the CPT manual, identify the following physical status modifiers:

9. Patient with a severe systemic disease that is a constant threat to life.

   Modifier: _____

10. Normal healthy patient.

    Modifier: _____

11. Patient with a severe systemic disease.

    Modifier: _____

12. Declared brain-dead patient whose organs are being removed for donor purposes.

    Modifier: _____

13. Patient with mild systemic disease.

    Modifier: _____

14. Moribund patient who is not expected to survive without the operation.

    Modifier: _____

Locate anesthesia procedures in the CPT manual index under the entry "Anesthesia" and then subtermed by the anatomic site. Write the CPT index location on the line provided (e.g., Anesthesia, Thyroid). Then locate the code identified in the anesthesia section of the CPT manual. Choose the correct code and write the code on the line provided.

15. Diagnostic arthroscopic procedure of knee joint.

    Index location: _____

    CPT Code: _____

16. Radical hysterectomy.

    Index location: _____

    CPT Code: _____

17. Corneal transplant.

    Index location: _____

    CPT Code: _____

Odd-numbered answers are located in Appendix B, while the full answer key is only available in the TEACH Instructor Resources on Evolve.

Copyright © 2016 by Elsevier Inc.

18. Cesarean delivery only.

    Index location: _____

    CPT Code: _____

19. Otoscopy used in procedure for middle ear.

    Index location: _____

    CPT Code: _____

20. Transurethral resection of the prostate.

    Index location: _____

    CPT Code: _____

21. Anesthesia for a cardiac catheterization patient having mild systemic disease.

    CPT Code: _____

22. Anesthesia for a myringotomy on a healthy 5-year-old patient.

    CPT Code: _____

Assign the diagnosis code(s) for Questions 23–26.

23. Diverticulitis of colon with hemorrhage.

    ICD-10-CM Code: _____

    (ICD-9-CM Code: _____)

24. Atherosclerosis of coronary artery bypass graft utilizing internal mammary artery.

    ICD-10-CM Code: _____

    (ICD-9-CM Code: _____)

25. Toxic diffuse goiter with thyrotoxic crisis.

    ICD-10-CM Code: _____

    (ICD-9-CM Code: _____)

26. Mitral valve regurgitation as a late effect of Fen-Phen, taken as prescribed, initial encounter.

    ICD-10-CM Codes: _____, _____

    (ICD-9-CM Codes: _____, _____)

Odd-numbered answers are located in Appendix B, while the full answer key is only available in the TEACH Instructor Resources on Evolve.

Copyright © 2016 by Elsevier Inc.

REPORTS

In Appendix A of this workbook you will find a section titled Reports, which contains original reports. Read the reports indicated below and supply the appropriate CPT anesthesia codes on the following lines:

27. Report 7

    CPT Code: _____

28. Report 41

    CPT Code: _____

29. Report 44

    CPT Code: _____

30. Report 83

    CPT Code: _____

Odd-numbered answers are located in Appendix B, while the full answer key is only available in the TEACH Instructor Resources on Evolve.

Copyright © 2016 by Elsevier Inc.

CHAPTER 13

Surgery Guidelines and General Surgery

THEORY

Without the use of reference material, answer the following:

1. The more complex subsections referred to in the text are Integumentary, Musculoskeletal, Respiratory, Cardiovascular, Digestive,

   and _____.

2. The information in the _____ contains information that is necessary to correctly code in the section, and the information is not repeated elsewhere.

3. Notes may appear before subsections, subheadings, _____, and subcategories within the CPT manual.

4. When a note is present, that note must be read and

   _____ if the coding is to be accurate.

5. Within the Surgery Guidelines, the _____ procedure codes are presented in a list by anatomic site.

6. According to the CPT manual, "Pertinent information [in the

   _____ report] should include an adequate definition or description of the nature, extent, need, time, effort, and equipment necessary to provide the service."

7. There are minor and _____ procedure designations for the purposes of a surgical package.

8. If a breast biopsy and mastectomy of the left breast were performed during the same operative session, would both procedures be reported?

   _____

9. If a breast biopsy and right knee operation were performed during the same operative session, would both procedures be reported?

   _____

Odd-numbered answers are located in Appendix B, while the full answer key is only available in the TEACH Instructor Resources on Evolve.

Copyright © 2016 by Elsevier Inc.

10. The CPT manual describes the surgical package as including one related preoperative E/M service, the operative procedure, and immediate

    _____ care.

11. Local infiltration is considered _____ anesthesia.

12. This term means a worsening as described in the text.

    _____

13. This type of anesthesia is not part of the surgical package.

    _____

14. The predefined number of days before and after a surgical procedure are

    referred to as the _____ period.

15. What is the CPT code that reports a surgical tray? _____

16. What is the HCPCS code that reports a surgical tray?

    _____

17. According to the Medicare guidelines, a surgical package includes the

    treatment of complications by the _____ physician.

18. At an office visit, a decision for surgery was made. The surgical procedure was scheduled 21 days later. Would the office visit service be:
    a. reported separately
    b. included in the surgical procedure

19. Splitting open of the surgical wound is _____.

20. Inclusion or exclusion of a procedure in the CPT manual implies health insurance coverage or no health insurance coverage.

    True or False? _____

Odd-numbered answers are located in Appendix B, while the full answer key is only available in the TEACH Instructor Resources on Evolve.

Copyright © 2016 by Elsevier Inc.

PRACTICAL

With the use of a CPT manual, answer the following:

21. The code range in the Surgical section is _____ to

_____.

22. The subsection that follows the Digestive System is the

_____ System.

23. What type of microscope has a subsection of the Surgery section?

_____

24. The difference between 10021 and 10022 is that one is with

_____ _____ and one is without it.

25. According to the parenthetical information following code 10022, for a percutaneous needle biopsy other than fine needle aspiration, see

_____ for salivary gland.

26. According to the Surgery Guidelines, codes designated as

" _____ _____ " should not be reported in addition to the code for the total procedure or service of which it is considered an integral component.

27. According to the Surgery Guidelines, follow-up care for

_____ surgical procedures includes only that care which is usually a part of the surgical procedure.

28. According to the Surgery Guidelines, the code range for Maternity Care

and Delivery is _____-_____.

29. According to the Surgery Guidelines, this is the code for unlisted

procedures of the lip. _____

30. According to the Surgery Guidelines, this is the code for unlisted

procedures of the urinary system. _____

Odd-numbered answers are located in Appendix B, while the full answer key is only available in the TEACH Instructor Resources on Evolve.

CHAPTER 14

Integumentary System

THEORY

Make sure to check
evolve
for the latest
content updates

Integumentary System Terminology

Match the following terms to the correct definitions:

1. ____ Dermis

2. ____ Epidermis

3. ____ Subcutaneous

4. ____ Incision and drainage

5. ____ Abscess

6. ____ Cyst

7. ____ Debridement

8. ____ Paring

9. ____ Biopsy

10. ____ Shaving

a. Localized collection of pus that will result in the disintegration of tissue over time

b. Second layer of skin holding blood vessels, nerve endings, sweat glands, and hair follicles

c. Removal of a small piece of living tissue for diagnostic purposes

d. Outer layer of skin

e. Horizontal or transverse removal of dermal or epidermal lesions, without full-thickness excision

f. Cleansing of or removing dead tissue from a wound

g. To cut and withdraw fluid

h. Removal of thin layers of skin by peeling or scraping

i. Tissue below dermis, primarily fat cells that insulate the body

j. Closed sac containing matter or fluid

Odd-numbered answers are located in Appendix B, while the full answer key is only available in the TEACH Instructor Resources on Evolve.

Copyright © 2016 by Elsevier Inc.

Match the following terms to the correct definitions:

11. _____ Excision

12. _____ Benign

13. _____ Malignant

14. _____ Repair

15. _____ Skin graft

16. _____ Tissue transfer

17. _____ Destruction

18. _____ Mast-

19. _____ Cryosurgery

a. Full-thickness removal of a lesion that may include simple closure

b. Prefix meaning breast

c. Transplantation of tissue to repair a defect

d. Not progressive or recurrent

e. Killing of tissue, possibly by electrocautery, laser, chemical, or other means

f. Destruction of lesions using extreme cold

g. Pertains to suturing a wound

h. Piece of skin for grafting that is still partially attached to the original blood supply and is used to cover an adjacent wound area

i. Used to describe a cancerous tumor that grows worse over time

20. If multiple lesions are treated, the most complex lesion is listed first and the others are usually listed using modifier:
    a. -50
    b. -51
    c. -47
    d. -99

21. This condition is chronic abscessing and subsequent infection of a sweat gland.
    a. folliculitis
    b. hyperhidrosis
    c. miliaria
    d. hidradenitis

22. An example of a corn or callus is a benign:
    a. hyperkeratotic skin lesion
    b. lipoma or dermatofibroma
    c. nevi or dysplastic nevi
    d. dermoid cyst or nevi or dysplastic nevi

Odd-numbered answers are located in Appendix B, while the full answer key is only available in the TEACH Instructor Resources on Evolve.

Copyright © 2016 by Elsevier Inc.

PRACTICAL

Using the CPT and ICD-10-CM/ICD-9-CM manuals, code the following services:

23. Joan, an established patient, comes into the office to have an intermediate repair of a 2.6 cm wound on her right arm. A surgical tray was used.

    CPT Codes: _____, _____

    ICD-10-CM Code: _____

    (ICD-9-CM Code: _____)

24. Rita, an established patient, has a 16.2 cm simple repair of the cheek. A surgical tray is used.

    CPT Codes: _____, _____

    ICD-10-CM Code: _____

    (ICD-9-CM Code: _____)

25. Lisa, an established patient, has a percutaneous biopsy with stereotactic image guidance for a left breast mass. A surgical tray was used. The pathology report later indicated a neoplasm of uncertain behavior.

    CPT Codes: _____, _____

    ICD-10-CM Code: _____

    (ICD-9-CM Code: _____)

26. What code would be used to report Mr. Jones's visit to Dr. Green 2 weeks after major surgery?

    CPT Code: _____ E/M code

    ICD-10-CM Code: _____ Z code

    (ICD-9-CM Code: _____)

27. Excision axillary hidradenitis, complex repair.

    CPT Code: _____

    ICD-10-CM Code: _____

    (ICD-9-CM Code: _____)

28. Debridement; 16 sq. cm. subcutaneous tissue and muscle due to a diabetic foot ulcer.

    CPT Code: _____

    ICD-10-CM Codes: _____, _____

    (ICD-9-CM Codes: _____, _____)

Odd-numbered answers are located in Appendix B, while the full answer key is only available in the TEACH Instructor Resources on Evolve.

Copyright © 2016 by Elsevier Inc.

29. Removal of tissue expander without insertion of prosthesis.

   CPT Code: _____

30. Excision of abscessed pilonidal cyst; complicated.

   CPT Code: _____

   ICD-10-CM Code: _____

   (ICD-9-CM Code: _____)

31. Removal of subdermal contraceptive implant.

   CPT Code: _____

   ICD-10-CM Code: _____

   (ICD-9-CM Code: _____)

32. Debridement of four fingernails due to onychomycosis.

   CPT Code: _____

   ICD-10-CM Code: _____

   (ICD-9-CM Code: _____)

33. Excision of 4 cm benign lesion of face (most resource intensive) and excision of 3 cm benign lesion of neck.

   🔗 CPT Code(s): _____

   🔗 ICD-10-CM Code(s): _____

   (🔗 ICD-9-CM Code(s): _____)

34. Excision of a 2.5 cm malignant lip lesion and two malignant lesions of the skin of the chest, each 1.5 cm in diameter.

   🔗 CPT Code(s): _____

   🔗 ICD-10-CM Code(s): _____

   (🔗 ICD-9-CM Code(s): _____)

35. Destruction by laser of three premalignant actinic keratoses facial lesions.

   🔗 CPT Code(s): _____

   🔗 ICD-10-CM Code(s): _____

   (🔗 ICD-9-CM Code(s): _____)

🔗 **User to decide number of codes necessary to correctly answer the question.**
Odd-numbered answers are located in Appendix B, while the full answer key is only available in the TEACH Instructor Resources on Evolve.

Copyright © 2016 by Elsevier Inc.

36. Destruction of 4.0 cm malignant lesion of the eyelid.

 🌀 CPT Code(s): _____

 🌀 ICD-10-CM Code(s): _____

 (🌀 ICD-9-CM Code(s): _____)

37. Suzanne Osterland, a 4-year-old, is brought to the office by her father. Suzanne was playing on the swing set at the playground when she fell approximately 5 feet from the top step of the play set. When she fell, she struck her leg on a birdbath rim and then on the playground gardener's pail with several garden forks protruding over the rim, sustaining 12.9 cm, 3.1 cm, and 2.1 cm lacerations of the lower right leg, requiring deep-layered closure accomplished after subcutaneous tissue debridement of 18 sq. cm.

 CPT Codes: _____, _____

 ICD-10-CM Codes: _____, _____ (W code),

 _____ (W code), _____ (Y code)

 (ICD-9-CM Codes: _____, _____ (E code),

 _____ (E code), _____ (E code),

 _____ (E code))

38. Electrosurgical destruction of a 1.0 cm malignant lesion of the neck.

 🌀 CPT Code(s): _____

 🌀 ICD-10-CM Code(s): _____

 (🌀 ICD-9-CM Code(s): _____)

39. Cryosurgical destruction of 10 flat warts on the hand.

 🌀 CPT Code(s): _____

 🌀 ICD-10-CM Code(s): _____

 (🌀 ICD-9-CM Code(s): _____)

40. Laser destruction of multiple malignant lesions, as follows: 3.4 cm on right hand, 2.1 cm on left hand, 5.2 cm on right hand, 4.3 cm on left hand, 0.3 cm on right eyelid, 0.5 cm on left eyelid.

 🌀 CPT Code(s): _____

 🌀 ICD-10-CM Code(s): _____

 (🌀 ICD-9-CM Code(s): _____)

🌀 User to decide number of codes necessary to correctly answer the question.
Odd-numbered answers are located in Appendix B, while the full answer key is only available in the TEACH Instructor Resources on Evolve.

Copyright © 2016 by Elsevier Inc.

41. Debridement of back for extensive eczematous skin, 20% body surface.

   🔘 CPT Code(s): _____

   🔘 ICD-10-CM Code(s): _____

   (🔘 ICD-9-CM Code(s): _____)

42. Bilateral blepharoplasty of upper eyelid due to ptosis.

   🔘 CPT Code(s): _____

   🔘 ICD-10-CM Code(s): _____

   (🔘 ICD-9-CM Code(s): _____)

43. Initial, local treatment, first-degree burn, of back of hand, 5% body surface. The burn was caused by steam from a pipe at his home that accidentally was connected improperly.

   🔘 CPT Code(s): _____

   🔘 ICD-10-CM Code(s): _____

   (🔘 ICD-9-CM Code(s): _____)

44. Mohs micrographic surgery of arm for a poorly defined malignant neoplasm, first stage, 4 tissue blocks.

   🔘 CPT Code(s): _____

   🔘 ICD-10-CM Code(s): _____

   (🔘 ICD-9-CM Code(s): _____)

45. Mastotomy with drainage of deep abscess.

   🔘 CPT Code(s): _____

   🔘 ICD-10-CM Code(s): _____

   (🔘 ICD-9-CM Code(s): _____)

🔘 User to decide number of codes necessary to correctly answer the question.

Odd-numbered answers are located in Appendix B, while the full answer key is only available in the TEACH Instructor Resources on Evolve.

Copyright © 2016 by Elsevier Inc.

REPORTS

In Appendix A of this workbook you will find a section titled Reports, which contains original reports. Read the reports indicated below and supply the appropriate CPT and ICD-10-CM/ICD-9-CM codes on the following lines:

46. Report 6

 CPT Code(s): _____

 ICD-10-CM Code(s): _____

 (ICD-9-CM Code(s): _____)

47. Report 7

 CPT Code(s): _____

 ICD-10-CM Code(s): _____

 (ICD-9-CM Code(s): _____)

48. Report 8

 CPT Code(s): _____

 ICD-10-CM Code(s): _____

 (ICD-9-CM Code(s): _____)

49. Report 9

 CPT Code(s): _____

 ICD-10-CM Code(s): _____

 (ICD-9-CM Code(s): _____)

50. Report 11

 CPT Code(s): _____

 ICD-10-CM Code(s): _____

 (ICD-9-CM Code(s): _____)

51. Report 12

 CPT Code(s): _____

 ICD-10-CM Code(s): _____

 (ICD-9-CM Code(s): _____)

 User to decide number of codes necessary to correctly answer the question.
Odd-numbered answers are located in Appendix B, while the full answer key is only available in the TEACH Instructor Resources on Evolve.

Copyright © 2016 by Elsevier Inc.

CHAPTER 15

Musculoskeletal System

THEORY

Make sure to check
evolve
for the latest
content updates

Musculoskeletal Terminology

Without the use of reference material, match the following terms to the correct definitions:

1. _____ Closed treatment

2. _____ Open treatment

3. _____ Percutaneous

4. _____ Fracture

5. _____ Dislocation

6. _____ Manipulation

7. _____ Fixation

8. _____ Skeletal traction

9. _____ Soft tissue

10. _____ Arthroplasty

11. _____ Arthrodesis

a. Application of force to a limb with the use of a pin, screw, wire, or clamp attached to the bone

b. Displacement of a bone from its normal location in a joint

c. The application of pins, wires, screws, and so on to immobilize; these can be placed externally or internally

d. Fracture treatment when site is not surgically opened and visualized or reduction

e. Word used interchangeably with reduction to mean the attempted restoration of a fracture or joint dislocation to its normal anatomic position

f. Fracture site that is surgically opened and visualized

g. Surgical immobilization of a joint

h. Tissues (fascia, connective tissue, muscle, etc.) surrounding organs and other structures

i. Break in a bone

j. Fixation considered neither open nor closed; fracture is not visualized, but fixation is placed across the fracture site under x-ray imaging

k. Reshaping or reconstructing a joint

Odd-numbered answers are located in Appendix B, while the full answer key is only available in the TEACH Instructor Resources on Evolve.

Copyright © 2016 by Elsevier Inc.

Without the use of reference material, answer the following:

12. Would a biopsy code usually include the administration of any necessary local anesthesia? Yes or No? _____

13. What is arthrocentesis? _____

14. What is a uniplane fixation device? _____

_____

15. What is the name of the graft that is taken from the upper thigh area

where the fascia is the thickest? _____

16. What type of stimulation often is used to promote healing of a slow-

healing fracture? _____

17. What is fast becoming the surgical method of choice for many

musculoskeletal procedures today? _____

18. What is the term that describes the use of tape applied to the body to

provide support or limit motion? _____

19. Do you bill for the removal of a cast that your physician applied?

Yes or No? _____ Why or why not? _____

_____

20. What two words describe when elastic wrap or tape is fastened to the skin or wrapped around a limb and weights are then attached to the

wraps or tape? _____

21. What is the primary difference between the excision codes found in the Musculoskeletal System subsection and the excision codes found in the

Integumentary System subsection? _____

_____

_____

Odd-numbered answers are located in Appendix B, while the full answer key is only available in the TEACH Instructor Resources on Evolve.

Copyright © 2016 by Elsevier Inc.

PRACTICAL

With the use of the CPT and ICD-10-CM/ICD-9-CM manual(s), code the following:

22. John is returning to the physician's office 2 weeks postsurgery for an application of a new long leg cast. The patient required surgery due to a traumatic fracture of the lower leg.

    CPT Code: _____

    ICD-10-CM Codes: _____, _____

    (ICD-9-CM Codes: _____, _____)

23. Julie Mason, age 5 years, is coming in today to have her long-arm cast removed and replaced with a short-arm cast for 3 weeks. The patient sustained a Torus fracture of the upper end of the radius and is 1 week postop.

    CPT Code: _____

    ICD-10-CM Codes: _____, _____

    (ICD-9-CM Codes: _____, _____)

24. Jamie Larson slipped on the ice and twisted her knee when she fell. During diagnostic arthroscopy, a bucket-handle tear of the medial and lateral meniscus was seen and repaired.

    CPT Code: _____

    ICD-10-CM Codes: _____, _____, _____

    (ICD-9-CM Codes: _____, _____,

    _____)

25. Percutaneous skeletal fixation of closed calcaneal fracture requiring manipulation.

    CPT Code: _____

    ICD-10-CM Code: _____

    (ICD-9-CM Code: _____)

Odd-numbered answers are located in Appendix B, while the full answer key is only available in the TEACH Instructor Resources on Evolve.

Copyright © 2016 by Elsevier Inc.

26. Closed treatment of multiple pelvic fractures without displacement of the pelvic ring; without manipulation.

    CPT Code: _____

    ICD-10-CM Code: _____

    (ICD-9-CM Code: _____)

27. Closed treatment of a single closed metacarpophalangeal dislocation, distal end; with manipulation and without anesthesia.

    CPT Code: _____

    ICD-10-CM Code: _____

    (ICD-9-CM Code: _____)

28. Open treatment of a closed traumatic anterior hip dislocation without fixation.

    CPT Code: _____

    ICD-10-CM Code: _____

    (ICD-9-CM Code: _____)

29. Closed treatment of a patellar fracture; no manipulation.

    CPT Code: _____

    ICD-10-CM Code: _____

    (ICD-9-CM Code: _____)

30. Closed treatment of a closed patellar dislocation; no anesthesia.

    CPT Code: _____

    ICD-10-CM Code: _____

    (ICD-9-CM Code: _____)

31. Manipulation of a knee joint under general anesthesia with application of a traction device. Patient had an anterior dislocation of the tibia, proximal end.

    CPT Code: _____

    ICD-10-CM Code: _____

    (ICD-9-CM Code: _____)

Odd-numbered answers are located in Appendix B, while the full answer key is only available in the TEACH Instructor Resources on Evolve.

Copyright © 2016 by Elsevier Inc.

32. Closed treatment of a closed tarsal bone dislocation without anesthesia.

    CPT Code: _____

    ICD-10-CM Code: _____

    (ICD-9-CM Code: _____)

33. Depressed frontal sinus fracture repaired using open treatment.

    CPT Code: _____

34. Open treatment of a Le Fort I maxillary fracture.

    CPT Code: _____

35. Aspiration and injection of a bone cyst.

    CPT Code: _____

36. Removal of deep screws from a repaired fracture. (The screws are fixation devices.)

    CPT Code: _____

37. Replantation of index finger, including sublimis tendon insertion, following a complete traumatic amputation. Code only the replantation service.

    CPT Code: _____

38. Costochondral cartilage graft.

    CPT Code: _____

39. Therapeutic injection of corticosteroids for medial nerve entrapment (CTS).

    CPT Code: _____

    ICD-10-CM Code: _____

    (ICD-9-CM Code: _____)

40. Aspiration of a shoulder joint.

    CPT Code: _____

41. Removal of a halo that was applied by another physician.

    CPT Code: _____

Odd-numbered answers are located in Appendix B, while the full answer key is only available in the TEACH Instructor Resources on Evolve.

Copyright © 2016 by Elsevier Inc.

42. Subsequent removal of a short-arm cast by the physician who applied the cast.

    CPT Code: _____

43. Closed treatment of a mandibular fracture without manipulation.

    CPT Code: _____

44. Application of a shoulder-to-hip body cast.

    CPT Code: _____

45. Wedging of a clubfoot cast.

    CPT Code: _____

46. Application of a short leg splint.

    CPT Code: _____

47. Strapping of a hip.

    CPT Code: _____

48. Application of a long-arm splint.

    CPT Code: _____

49. Strapping of a 40-year-old's thorax.

    CPT Code: _____

50. Surgical arthroscopy of the temporomandibular joint.

    CPT Code: _____

51. Application, cast; figure-of-eight.

    CPT Code: _____

52. Surgical arthroscopy, elbow; limited debridement.

    CPT Code: _____

53. Diagnostic hip arthroscopy.

    CPT Code: _____

54. Surgical arthroscopy with lateral meniscus repair of knee.

    CPT Code: _____

Odd-numbered answers are located in Appendix B, while the full answer key is only available in the TEACH Instructor Resources on Evolve.

Copyright © 2016 by Elsevier Inc.

55. Arthroscopic chondroplasty of knee with minimal debridement.

    CPT Code: _____

56. Endoscopic plantar fasciotomy.

    CPT Code: _____

57. Release of a transverse carpal ligament of the wrist with surgical endoscopy.

    CPT Code: _____

58. Arthrocentesis of ganglion cyst of toe joint, both injection and aspiration.

    CPT Code: _____

    ICD-10-CM Code: _____

    (ICD-9-CM Code: _____)

59. Excision of maxillary torus palatinus.

    CPT Code: _____

Odd-numbered answers are located in Appendix B, while the full answer key is only available in the TEACH Instructor Resources on Evolve.

REPORTS

In Appendix A of this workbook you will find a section titled Reports, which contains original reports. Read the reports indicated below and supply the appropriate CPT and ICD-10-CM/ICD-9-CM codes on the following lines:

60. Report 10

   CPT Code: _____

   ICD-10-CM Codes: _____, _____,

   _____ (External Cause code)

   (ICD-9-CM Codes: _____, _____ (E code))

61. Report 13

   CPT Code: _____

   ICD-10-CM Code: _____

   (ICD-9-CM Code: _____)

62. Report 14

   CPT Code: _____

   ICD-10-CM Codes: _____, _____

   (ICD-9-CM Codes: _____, _____)

63. Report 15

   CPT Code: _____

   ICD-10-CM Codes: _____, _____

   (ICD-9-CM Codes: _____, _____)

64. Report 16

   CPT Code: _____

   ICD-10-CM Codes: _____, _____

   (ICD-9-CM Codes: _____, _____)

Odd-numbered answers are located in Appendix B, while the full answer key is only available in the TEACH Instructor Resources on Evolve.

Copyright © 2016 by Elsevier Inc.

65. Report 17

   CPT Code: _____

   ICD-10-CM Code: _____

   (ICD-9-CM Codes: _____, _____)

66. Report 18

   CPT Code: _____

   ICD-10-CM Code: _____

   (ICD-9-CM Code: _____)

Odd-numbered answers are located in Appendix B, while the full answer key is only available in the TEACH Instructor Resources on Evolve.

Copyright © 2016 by Elsevier Inc.

CHAPTER 16

Respiratory System

THEORY

Without the use of reference material, complete the following:

Respiratory Terminology

Match the following terms and prefixes to the correct definitions:

1. _____ Polyp
2. _____ Rhino-
3. _____ Endoscopy
4. _____ Sinuses
5. _____ Antrum
6. _____ Antrotomy
7. _____ Laryngo-
8. _____ Bronchoscopy
9. _____ Thoracentesis
10. _____ Thoracotomy
11. _____ Thoracostomy
12. _____ Thoracoscopy
13. _____ Lobectomy
14. _____ Pleura
15. _____ Pneumo-
16. _____ Embolectomy

a. Excision of a lobe of the lung
b. Maxillary sinus
c. Prefix meaning larynx
d. Tumor on a pedicle that bleeds easily and may become malignant
e. Prefix meaning lung or air
f. Surgical puncture of the thoracic cavity, usually using a needle, to remove fluids
g. Inspection of the bronchial tree using a bronchoscope
h. Prefix meaning nose
i. Use of a lighted endoscope to view the pleural spaces and thoracic cavity or perform surgical procedures
j. Removal of blockage (embolism) from vessels
k. Inspection of body organs or cavities using a lighted scope that may be placed through an existing opening or through a small incision
l. Covering of the lungs and thoracic cavity that is moistened with serous fluid to reduce friction during respiratory movements of the lungs
m. Cutting into the thoracic cavity to allow for enlargement of the heart or for drainage
n. Cutting through the antrum wall to make an opening in the sinus
o. Cavities within the nasal bones
p. Surgical incision into the thoracic cavity

Odd-numbered answers are located in Appendix B, while the full answer key is only available in the TEACH Instructor Resources on Evolve.

Copyright © 2016 by Elsevier Inc.

17. What is the name of the item that is placed into the hole in a deviated septum as a repair without surgical grafting?

_____

18. What is the name of the surgical procedure for the reshaping of the nose?

_____

19. What is the name of the surgical procedure for the rearrangement of the nasal septum often used in patients with a deviated septum?

_____

20. This term means destruction by removing, usually by vaporization, chipping, or other erosive process such as laser or cutting:

_____

21. Which approach of treating nasal hemorrhage is most difficult to control, posterior or anterior?

_____

22. What term describes washing out of an organ?

_____

23. What are the two different approaches that can be used to perform a

tracheostomy? _____ and _____

24. If a surgeon performs a thoracotomy procedure and at the end of the procedure inserts a chest tube for drainage, do you report the insertion of the tube separately? Why?

_____

25. If bilateral destruction of maxillary sinuses is performed, what modifier

would you use? _____

26. Removal of two lobes of a lung is termed a(n)

_____.

Odd-numbered answers are located in Appendix B, while the full answer key is only available in the TEACH Instructor Resources on Evolve.

Copyright © 2016 by Elsevier Inc.

PRACTICAL

With the use of the CPT and ICD-10-CM/ICD-9-CM manuals, complete the following:

27. Endoscopic maxillary antrostomy with removal of granulation tissue.

    CPT Code: _____

28. Ben is a 5-year-old who swallowed a nickel. Patient needed an indirect laryngoscopy to remove this foreign body.

    CPT Code: _____

29. Bronchoscopy with transbronchial biopsies of two lobes of the right lung.

    CPT Codes: _____, _____

30. Flexible bronchoscopy with brushings.

    CPT Code: _____

31. Diagnostic flexible fiberoptic laryngoscopy.

    CPT Code: _____

32. Intranasal biopsy.

    CPT Code: _____

33. Cauterization of superficial mucosa of bilateral inferior turbinates.

    CPT Code: _____

34. Primary rhinoplasty with elevation of nasal tip.

    CPT Code: _____

35. Extensive bilateral removal of nasal polyps, performed in the hospital outpatient department.

    CPT Codes: _____, _____

36. Insertion of a septal button.

    CPT Code: _____

37. Direct, operative, laryngoscopy with biopsy, with use of the operating microscope.

    CPT Code: _____

Odd-numbered answers are located in Appendix B, while the full answer key is only available in the TEACH Instructor Resources on Evolve.

38. Establishment and subsequent insertion of voice button following construction of a transesophageal fistula.

    CPT Code: _____

39. Arytenoidectomy; external approach.

    CPT Code(s): _____

40. Laryngoscopy, with stroboscopy.

    CPT Code(s): _____

41. Nasotracheal catheter aspiration.

    CPT Code(s): _____

42. Cervical tracheoplasty.

    CPT Code(s): _____

43. Revision of a tracheostomy scar.

    CPT Code(s): _____

44. Thoracentesis for aspiration of the pleural space, without image guidance.

    CPT Code(s): _____

45. Surgical thoracoscopy, with removal of a clot from pericardial.

    CPT Code(s): _____

46. Double lung transplant with cardiopulmonary bypass.

    CPT Code(s): _____

47. Repair hernia of the lung through the chest wall.

    CPT Code(s): _____

48. Open closure of a major bronchial fistula.

    CPT Code(s): _____

49. Therapeutic fracture of inferior nasal turbinate bone, closed.

    CPT Code(s): _____

User to decide number of codes necessary to correctly answer the question.
Odd-numbered answers are located in Appendix B, while the full answer key is only available in the TEACH Instructor Resources on Evolve.

Copyright © 2016 by Elsevier Inc.

50. Sinusotomy, sphenoid, without biopsy for acute sinusitis.

    🔾 CPT Code(s): _____

    🔾 ICD-10-CM Code(s): _____

    (🔾 ICD-9-CM Code(s): _____)

51. Tracheostoma revision, simple, without flap rotation due to infection of tracheostomy by cellulitis.

    🔾 CPT Code(s): _____

    🔾 ICD-10-CM Code(s): _____

    (🔾 ICD-9-CM Code(s): _____)

52. Bronchial biopsy, bronchoscopic, due to chronic cough.

    🔾 CPT Code(s): _____

    🔾 ICD-10-CM Code(s): _____

    (🔾 ICD-9-CM Code(s): _____)

53. Total pneumonectomy due to occupational asbestosis.

    🔾 CPT Code(s): _____

    🔾 ICD-10-CM Code(s): _____

    (🔾 ICD-9-CM Code(s): _____)

54. Diagnostic thoracoscopy of the pericardial sac, with biopsy for chronic rheumatic pericarditis.

    🔾 CPT Code(s): _____

    🔾 ICD-10-CM Code(s): _____

    (🔾 ICD-9-CM Code(s): _____)

55. Extrapleural resection of the ribs, all stages for deformed ribs, congenital.

    🔾 CPT Code(s): _____

    🔾 ICD-10-CM Code(s): _____

    (🔾 ICD-9-CM Code(s): _____)

🔾 **User to decide number of codes necessary to correctly answer the question.**
Odd-numbered answers are located in Appendix B, while the full answer key is only available in the TEACH Instructor Resources on Evolve.

Copyright © 2016 by Elsevier Inc.

56. Carinal reconstruction for lung cancer, primary, malignant.

    ⊛ CPT Code(s): _____

    ⊛ ICD-10-CM Code(s): _____

    (⊛ ICD-9-CM Code(s): _____)

57. Instillation, via a catheter, of an agent for pleurodesis for malignant pleural effusion due to ovarian cancer.

    ⊛ CPT Code(s): _____

    ⊛ ICD-10-CM Code(s): _____

    (⊛ ICD-9-CM Code(s): _____)

58. Excision dermoid cyst of the nose, complex.

    ⊛ CPT Code(s): _____

    ⊛ ICD-10-CM Code(s): _____

    (⊛ ICD-9-CM Code(s): _____)

⊛ User to decide number of codes necessary to correctly answer the question.
Odd-numbered answers are located in Appendix B, while the full answer key is only available in the TEACH Instructor Resources on Evolve.

Copyright © 2016 by Elsevier Inc.

REPORTS

In Appendix A of this workbook you will find a section titled Reports, which contains original reports. Read the reports indicated below and supply the appropriate CPT and ICD-10-CM/ICD-9-CM codes on the following lines:

59. Report 19

    ✪ CPT Code(s): _____

    ✪ ICD-10-CM Code(s): _____

    (✪ ICD-9-CM Code(s): _____)

60. Report 21

    ✪ CPT Code(s): _____

    ✪ ICD-10-CM Code(s): _____

    (✪ ICD-9-CM Code(s): _____)

61. Report 23

    ✪ CPT Code(s): _____

    ✪ ICD-10-CM Code(s): _____

    (✪ ICD-9-CM Code(s): _____)

62. Report 24

    ✪ CPT Code(s): _____

    ✪ ICD-10-CM Code(s): _____

    (✪ ICD-9-CM Code(s): _____)

✪ **User to decide number of codes necessary to correctly answer the question.**
Odd-numbered answers are located in Appendix B, while the full answer key is only available in the TEACH Instructor Resources on Evolve.

CHAPTER 17

Cardiovascular System

THEORY

Cardiovascular Terminology

Without the use of reference material, match the following terms to the correct definitions:

1. _____ Pericardium

2. _____ Cardiopulmonary

3. _____ Bypass

4. _____ Pacemaker

5. _____ Single-chamber device

6. _____ Dual-chamber device

7. _____ Electrode

8. _____ Ventricle

9. _____ Atrium

10. _____ Implantable defibrillator

11. _____ Artery

a. Lead attached to a generator that carries the electrical current from the generator to the atria or ventricles

b. To go around

c. Surgically placed device that directs an electrical current shock to the heart to restore rhythm

d. Electrode of the pacemaker is placed only in the atrium or only in the ventricle, but not in both places

e. Membranous sac enclosing the heart and ends of the great vessels

f. Vessel that carries oxygenated blood from the heart to the body tissues

g. Refers to the heart and lungs

h. Electrodes of the pacemaker are placed in both the right atrium and the right ventricle of the heart

i. Chamber in the upper part of the heart

j. Electrical device that controls the beating of the heart by electrical impulses

k. Chamber in the lower part of the heart

Odd-numbered answers are located in Appendix B, while the full answer key is only available in the TEACH Instructor Resources on Evolve.

Copyright © 2016 by Elsevier Inc.

Match the following terms to the correct definitions:

12. _____ Vein

13. _____ Aneurysm

14. _____ Embolism

15. _____ Thrombosis

16. _____ Endarterectomy

17. _____ Angioplasty

18. _____ Injection

19. _____ Catheter

20. _____ Arteriovenous fistula

21. _____ Anomaly

22. _____ Ischemia

23. _____ Cardiopulmonary bypass

24. _____ Fistula

25. _____ Shunt

a. Forcing of fluid into a vessel or cavity

b. Blood bypasses the heart through a heart-lung machine during open heart surgery

c. Vessel that carries deoxygenated blood to the heart from the body tissues

d. Blood clot

e. Abnormal opening from one area to another area within the body or to outside of the body

f. Blockage of a blood vessel by a blood clot or other matter that has moved from another area of the body through the circulatory system

g. Direct communication (passage) between an artery and vein

h. Tube placed into the body to put fluid in or take fluid out

i. Surgical or percutaneous procedure on a vessel to dilate the vessel open, used in treatment of atherosclerotic disease

j. A sac of clotted blood or fluid formed in the circulatory system (e.g., vein or artery)

k. Incision into an artery to remove the inner lining to remove disease or blockage

l. Divert or make an artificial passage

m. Deficient blood supply caused by obstruction of the circulatory system

n. Abnormality

26. The term that describes the procedure in which the surgeon withdraws fluid from the pericardial space by means of a needle inserted into the

space is _____.

Odd-numbered answers are located in Appendix B, while the full answer key is only available in the TEACH Instructor Resources on Evolve.

Copyright © 2016 by Elsevier Inc.

27. Codes for excision of cardiac tumors are divided based on whether the

    tumor is located _____ or _____.

28. What are the names of two devices that are inserted into the body to

    electrically shock the heart into regular rhythm? _____

    and _____

29. The two approaches used to insert devices that electrically shock the

    heart into regular rhythm are _____ and

    _____.

30. If the patient is returned to the operating room for repositioning or
    replacement of the pacemaker or implantable defibrillator during the

    global period, modifier _____ would be appended to the code.

31. If a physician implanted a pacemaker and 10 days later the patient
    returns to the same surgeon for removal of sutures, would you charge
    for the service? Why?

    _____, _____

32. If a patient is seen for a rash on the heel of the foot by the same
    physician who implanted a pacemaker 20 days earlier, would you bill

    for the office service for the rash? _____

33. When you bill for E/M services unrelated to a pacemaker implantation
    during the allowable follow-up days, what modifier would you use on

    the code to alert the third-party payer? _____

34. What are the four cardiac valves? _____,

    _____, _____, and _____

35. What is the name of the device that can be surgically implanted into
    the subcutaneous tissue in the upper left quadrant to record heart
    rhythms when the patient depresses a button?

    _____

36. What arteries feed the heart? _____

37. When a heart artery is clogged and the heart muscle performs at a low
    level as a result of a lack of blood, the condition is called

    _____ ischemia.

**Odd-numbered answers are located in Appendix B, while the full answer key is only available in the TEACH
Instructor Resources on Evolve.**

Copyright © 2016 by Elsevier Inc.

38. When a heart artery is clogged and the heart muscle dies, the condition

is called _____ ischemia.

39. A mass of undissolved matter in the blood that is transported by the

blood current is a(n) _____.

40. Local anesthesia, catheter introduction, and injection of

_____ _____ are procedures that are
included in a vascular injection.

Odd-numbered answers are located in Appendix B, while the full answer key is only available in the TEACH Instructor Resources on Evolve.

106

Copyright © 2016 by Elsevier Inc.

PRACTICAL

Using the CPT and ICD-10-CM/ICD-9-CM manuals, code the following:

41. Valvuloplasty of the aortic valve using transventricular dilation with cardiopulmonary bypass.

    CPT Code: _____

42. Replacement aortic valve, with cardiopulmonary bypass, with prosthetic valve.

    CPT Code: _____

43. Valvuloplasty, tricuspid valve, with ring insertion.

    CPT Code: _____

44. Repair of a coronary arteriovenous fistula, without cardiopulmonary bypass.

    CPT Code: _____

45. Routine ECG with 12 leads with both the professional and technical components.

    CPT Code: _____

46. External electrical cardioversion.

    CPT Code: _____

47. Percutaneous balloon angioplasty; one coronary vessel.

    CPT Code: _____

48. CPR (Cardiopulmonary resuscitation).

    CPT Code: _____

49. Electrocardiogram with interpretation and report only.

    CPT Code: _____

50. Bypass graft of the common carotid-ipsilateral internal carotid artery using synthetic vein.

    CPT Code: _____

51. Ligation of temporal artery.

    CPT Code: _____

Odd-numbered answers are located in Appendix B, while the full answer key is only available in the TEACH Instructor Resources on Evolve.

Copyright © 2016 by Elsevier Inc.

52. Ligation of a common iliac vein.

    CPT Code: _____

53. Open transluminal balloon angioplasty aorta.

    CPT Code: _____

54. Coronary artery bypass, single artery, for coronary atherosclerosis of native coronary artery in a transplanted heart.

    CPT Code: _____

    ICD-10-CM Code: _____

    (ICD-9-CM Code: _____)

55. Coronary artery bypass, four veins, no arteries. Diagnosis of acute coronary insufficiency.

    ⊛ CPT Code(s): _____

    ⊛ ICD-10-CM Code(s): _____

    (⊛ ICD-9-CM Code(s): _____)

56. Repair of injury to intra-abdominal blood vessel, inferior vena cava, hepatic vein, with a vein graft.

    ⊛ CPT Code(s): _____

    ⊛ ICD-10-CM Code(s): _____

    (⊛ ICD-9-CM Code(s): _____)

57. Percutaneous insertion of an intra-aortic balloon assist device due to initial episode of acute myocardial infarction and cardiogenic shock.

    ⊛ CPT Code(s): _____

    ⊛ ICD-10-CM Code(s): _____

    (⊛ ICD-9-CM Code(s): _____)

58. Repair of a traumatic arteriovenous fistula of a lower extremity.

    ⊛ CPT Code(s): _____

    ⊛ ICD-10-CM Code(s): _____

    (⊛ ICD-9-CM Code(s): _____)

⊛ User to decide number of codes necessary to correctly answer the question.
Odd-numbered answers are located in Appendix B, while the full answer key is only available in the TEACH Instructor Resources on Evolve.

Copyright © 2016 by Elsevier Inc.

59. Repair congenital atrial septal defect, secundum, with bypass and patch.

    🔗 CPT Code(s): _____

    🔗 ICD-10-CM Code(s): _____

    (🔗 ICD-9-CM Code(s): _____)

60. Repair of a patent ductus arteriosus by division on a 16-year-old patient.

    🔗 CPT Code(s): _____

    🔗 ICD-10-CM Code(s): _____

    (🔗 ICD-9-CM Code(s): _____)

61. Reoperation of one arterial coronary bypass graft and one vein bypass graft for arteriosclerosis of native arteries, 3 months following the initial procedure.

    🔗 CPT Code(s): _____

    🔗 ICD-10-CM Code(s): _____

    (🔗 ICD-9-CM Code(s): _____)

🔗 **User to decide number of codes necessary to correctly answer the question.**
Odd-numbered answers are located in Appendix B, while the full answer key is only available in the TEACH Instructor Resources on Evolve.

Copyright © 2016 by Elsevier Inc.

REPORTS

In Appendix A of this workbook you will find a section titled Reports, which contains original reports. Read the reports indicated below and supply the appropriate CPT and ICD-10-CM/ICD-9-CM codes on the following lines:

62. Report 25

   🔵 CPT Code(s): _____

   🔵 ICD-10-CM Code(s): _____

   (🔵 ICD-9-CM Code(s): _____)

63. Report 26

   🔵 CPT Code(s): _____

   🔵 ICD-10-CM Code(s): _____

   (🔵 ICD-9-CM Code(s): _____)

64. Report 27

   🔵 CPT Code(s): _____

   🔵 ICD-10-CM Code(s): _____

   (🔵 ICD-9-CM Code(s): _____)

🔵 **User to decide number of codes necessary to correctly answer the question.**
Odd-numbered answers are located in Appendix B, while the full answer key is only available in the TEACH Instructor Resources on Evolve.

Copyright © 2016 by Elsevier Inc.

CHAPTER 18

Hemic, Lymphatic, Mediastinum, and Diaphragm

THEORY

Make sure to check
evolve
for the latest
content updates

Hemic and Lymphatic Terminology

Without the use of reference material, match the following terms to the correct definitions:

1. _____ Axillary nodes

2. _____ Splenectomy

3. _____ Splenoportography

4. _____ Allogenic

5. _____ Thoracic duct

6. _____ Retroperitoneal

7. _____ Jugular nodes

8. _____ Cystic hygroma

9. _____ Cloquet's node

10. _____ Inguinofemoral

11. _____ Cannulation

12. _____ Abscess

a. Behind the sac holding the abdominal organs and viscera (peritoneum)

b. Excision of the spleen

c. Insertion of a tube into a duct or cavity

d. Lymph nodes located next to the large vein in the neck

e. Radiographic procedure to allow visualization of the splenic and portal veins of the spleen

f. Of the same species, but genetically different

g. Collection and distribution point for lymph and the largest lymph vessel located in the chest

h. Congenital deformity or benign tumor of the lymphatic system

i. Also called a gland; it is the highest of the deep groin lymph nodes

j. Term that refers to the groin and thigh

k. Lymph nodes located in the armpit

l. Localization of pus

Odd-numbered answers are located in Appendix B, while the full answer key is only available in the TEACH Instructor Resources on Evolve.

Match the following terms to the correct definitions:

13. _____	Autologous, autogenous	a.	Grafting of tissue from one source to another
14. _____	Aspiration	b.	Immature blood cells
15. _____	Stem cell	c.	Incision into a lymphatic vessel
16. _____	Transplantation	d.	Inflammation of a lymph node
17. _____	Lymph node	e.	Excision of a lymph node (or nodes)
18. _____	Lymphadenitis	f.	From oneself
19. _____	Lymphangiotomy	g.	Use of a needle and syringe to withdraw fluid
20. _____	Lymphadenectomy	h.	Station along the lymphatic system

Mediastinum and Diaphragm Terminology

Match the following terms to the correct definitions:

21. _____	Mediastinum	a.	Overlapping
22. _____	Diaphragm	b.	Surgical separation of the vagus nerve
23. _____	Mediastinotomy	c.	Muscular wall that separates the thoracic and abdominal cavities
24. _____	Fundoplasty	d.	Incision and repair of the pyloric channel
25. _____	Pyloroplasty		
26. _____	Diaphragmatic hernia	e.	Operation on the stomach for repair or reconfiguration
27. _____	Mediastinoscopy	f.	Repair of the bottom of an organ or muscle
28. _____	Imbrication	g.	Hernia that is near the esophagus
29. _____	Transthoracic	h.	Hernia of the diaphragm
30. _____	Transabdominal	i.	Across the abdomen
31. _____	Paraesophageal hiatus hernia	j.	Cutting into the mediastinum
32. _____	Gastroplasty	k.	Across the thorax
33. _____	Vagotomy	l.	Use of an endoscope inserted through a small incision to view the mediastinum
		m.	The area between the lungs that contains the heart, aorta, trachea, lymph nodes, thymus gland, esophagus, and bronchial tubes

Odd-numbered answers are located in Appendix B, while the full answer key is only available in the TEACH Instructor Resources on Evolve.

Copyright © 2016 by Elsevier Inc.

PRACTICAL

Using the CPT and ICD-10-CM/ICD-9-CM manuals, code the following:

34. Injection procedure for identification of the sentinel node with intradermal radioisotope injection for the staging of clinically negative axillae in a patient with primary, malignant neoplasm of the central portion of the right breast.

    🔵 CPT Code(s): _____

    🔵 ICD-10-CM Code(s): _____

    (🔵 ICD-9-CM Code(s): _____)

35. Radical cervical lymphadenectomy for patient with malignant primary cancer of the nipple of the left breast. Pathology findings of the lymphadenectomy were positive.

    🔵 CPT Code(s): _____

    🔵 ICD-10-CM Code(s): _____

    (🔵 ICD-9-CM Code(s): _____)

36. Drainage of an extensive lymph node abscess. Pathology report indicated *Staphylococcus*.

    🔵 CPT Code(s): _____

    🔵 ICD-10-CM Code(s): _____

    (🔵 ICD-9-CM Code(s): _____)

37. Autologous bone marrow transplantation for a patient who has acute myelogenous leukemia that has not shown any signs of remission.

    🔵 CPT Code(s): _____

    🔵 ICD-10-CM Code(s): _____

    (🔵 ICD-9-CM Code(s): _____)

38. Partial splenectomy for a 3-year-old child with sickle cell disease, Hb-C with crisis.

    CPT Code: _____

    ICD-10-CM Code: _____

    (ICD-9-CM Code: _____)

🔵 **User to decide number of codes necessary to correctly answer the question.**
Odd-numbered answers are located in Appendix B, while the full answer key is only available in the TEACH Instructor Resources on Evolve.

Copyright © 2016 by Elsevier Inc.

39. Harvesting of bone marrow for transplantation from a father for subsequent transplantation into the daughter. Report only the harvesting service.

    CPT Code: _____

    ICD-10-CM Code: _____

    (ICD-9-CM Code: _____)

40. Repair of laceration of diaphragm by means of abdominal approach.

    CPT Code: _____

41. Excision of mediastinal cyst.

    CPT Code: _____

42. Resection of diaphragm with simple repair.

    CPT Code: _____

43. Preparation of stem (hematopoietic progenitor) cells for transplantation that included thawing of previously frozen cells and washing of the cells.

    CPT Code: _____

44. Laparoscopic removal of the spleen.

    CPT Code: _____

45. A radiologist performs lymphoscintigraphy in the radiology department. A few hours later, the patient is taken to the operating room where the general surgeon injects blue dye into the internal mammary lymph node and then excises a sentinel lymph node.

    CPT Codes: _____-26 (for performing both the injection and imaging of the radioisotope in the radiology department [nuclear

    medicine, lymph nodes]), _____-59 (for injecting the

    blue dye), and _____ (for excision of the sentinel lymph node in the operating room)

Odd-numbered answers are located in Appendix B, while the full answer key is only available in the TEACH Instructor Resources on Evolve.

Copyright © 2016 by Elsevier Inc.

REPORT

In Appendix A of this workbook you will find a section titled Reports, which contains original reports. Read the report indicated below and supply the appropriate CPT and ICD-10-CM/ICD-9-CM codes on the following lines:

46. Report 89

        CPT Code: _____

        ICD-10-CM Codes: _____,

        _____ (External Cause code for how accident occurred),

        _____ (Y Code)

        (ICD-9-CM Codes: _____, _____
        (E code for how accident occurred))

Odd-numbered answers are located in Appendix B, while the full answer key is only available in the TEACH Instructor Resources on Evolve.

Copyright © 2016 by Elsevier Inc.

CHAPTER 19

Digestive System

THEORY

Make sure to check
evolve
for the latest
content updates

Digestive Terminology

Without the use of reference material, match the following terms to the correct definitions:

1. _____ Gloss-

2. _____ Gastro-

3. _____ Anastomosis

4. _____ Hernia

5. _____ Gastrointestinal

6. _____ Ostomy

7. _____ Colostomy

8. _____ Ileostomy

9. _____ Jejunostomy

a. Artificial opening between the colon and the abdominal wall

b. Prefix meaning tongue

c. Organ or tissue protruding through the wall or cavity that usually contains it

d. Prefix meaning stomach

e. Artificial opening between the ileum and the abdominal wall

f. Surgical connection of two tubular structures, such as two pieces of the intestine

g. Pertaining to the stomach and intestine

h. Artificial opening

i. Artificial opening between the jejunum and the abdominal wall

Odd-numbered answers are located in Appendix B, while the full answer key is only available in the TEACH Instructor Resources on Evolve.

Copyright © 2016 by Elsevier Inc.

Without reference material, match the following terms to the correct definitions:

10. _____ Gastrostomy

11. _____ Proctosigmoidoscopy

12. _____ Sigmoidoscopy

13. _____ Colonoscopy

14. _____ Cholangiography

15. _____ Chole-

16. _____ Hepat-

17. _____ Incarcerated

18. _____ Reducible

a. Regarding hernias, a constricted, irreducible hernia that may cause obstruction of an intestine

b. Artificial opening between the stomach and the abdominal wall

c. Radiographic recording of the bile ducts

d. Able to be corrected or put back into a normal position

e. Endoscopic examination of the entire colon that may include part of the terminal ileum

f. Prefix meaning liver

g. Endoscopic examination of the entire rectum and sigmoid colon that may include a portion of the descending colon

h. Prefix meaning bile

i. Endoscopic examination of the sigmoid colon and rectum

Odd-numbered answers are located in Appendix B, while the full answer key is only available in the TEACH Instructor Resources on Evolve.

Copyright © 2016 by Elsevier Inc.

PRACTICAL

Using the CPT and ICD-10-CM/ICD-9-CM manuals, code the following:

19. Rigid esophagoscopy with removal of a foreign body.

    CPT Code: _____

20. Ligation of an intraoral salivary duct.

    CPT Code: _____

21. Transection of esophagus with repair of esophageal varices.

    CPT Code: _____

22. Enterotomy of the small intestine for removal of a foreign body.

    CPT Code: _____

23. Complicated revision of a colostomy.

    CPT Code: _____

24. Frenotomy, labial.

    CPT Code: _____

25. Excision of a palate lesion without closure.

    CPT Code: _____

26. Removal of a foreign body from the pharynx.

    CPT Code: _____

27. Amy is an 18-year-old with severe snoring. She is having an adenoidectomy in order to treat her snoring.

    CPT Code: _____

28. Partial colectomy with colostomy.

    CPT Code: _____

29. Open repair of an incarcerated recurrent inguinal hernia.

    CPT Code: _____

30. Surgical laparoscopic placement of a gastric band.

    CPT Code: _____

Odd-numbered answers are located in Appendix B, while the full answer key is only available in the TEACH Instructor Resources on Evolve.

Copyright © 2016 by Elsevier Inc.

31. Full-thickness repair of the vermilion of the lip.

   CPT Code: _____

32. Simple repair of 1.6-cm laceration of floor of mouth.

   CPT Code: _____

33. Bilateral parotid duct diversion.

   CPT Code: _____

34. Surgical laparoscopic repair of a paraesophageal hernia with fundoplasty with implantation of mesh.

   CPT Code: _____

35. Biopsy of the stomach by laparotomy.

   CPT Code: _____

36. Nontube open ileostomy.

   CPT Code: _____

37. Colorrhaphy for multiple perforations of large intestine sustained in auto accident. No colostomy was required.

   CPT Code: _____

38. Incision and drainage of perirectal abscess.

   CPT Code: _____

39. Diagnostic abdominal laparoscopy.

   CPT Code: _____

40. PREPROCEDURE DIAGNOSIS: Screening colonoscopy.

   POSTPROCEDURE DIAGNOSIS: Colon polyps.

   PREMEDICATIONS: Fentanyl 100 mcg and Versed 4 mg.

   PROCEDURE: A colonoscopy was performed to the cecum. The scope was advanced to the cecum under direct vision without any difficulty.

   FINDINGS: The cecum, ascending, transverse, descending, and sigmoid colon was normal. In the descending colon, there was a 2-mm polyp that was biopsied and submitted for histology.

   ASSESSMENT: Diminutive colon polyps.

Odd-numbered answers are located in Appendix B, while the full answer key is only available in the TEACH Instructor Resources on Evolve.

Copyright © 2016 by Elsevier Inc.

Pathology Report later indicated benign polyps.

CPT Code: _____

ICD-10-CM Codes: _____, _____

(ICD-9-CM Codes: _____, _____)

41. The patient presented to the emergency department complaining of vomiting coffee-ground material several times within the past 2 hours. He has abdominal pain and has been unable to eat for the past 24 hours. He is dizzy and light-headed. Two stools today have been black and tarry. While in the emergency department, he vomited bright-red blood and some coffee-ground material. A nasogastric tube was inserted and attached to suction with fluoro. An abdominal exam showed a fluid wave consistent with ascites. An IV of lactated ringers was started, and CBC and clotting studies were drawn. A detailed history and physical exam with high-complexity medical decision making were documented. A GI consultant was called and the patient was taken to Endoscopy for further evaluation of upper GI bleeding. Diagnosis: hematemesis, rule out esophageal varices; blood loss anemia (CBC review) acute; ascites. Code the services of the ED physician.

CPT Codes: _____, _____

ICD-10-CM Codes: _____, _____, _____

(ICD-9-CM Codes: _____, _____,

_____)

Odd-numbered answers are located in Appendix B, while the full answer key is only available in the TEACH Instructor Resources on Evolve.

REPORTS

In Appendix A of this workbook you will find a section titled Reports, which contains original reports. Read the reports indicated below and supply the appropriate CPT and ICD-10-CM/ICD-9-CM codes on the following lines:

42. Report 22

   🔘 CPT Code(s): _____

   🔘 ICD-10-CM Code(s): _____

   (🔘 ICD-9-CM Code(s): _____)

43. Report 31

   🔘 CPT Code(s): _____

   🔘 ICD-10-CM Code(s): _____

   (🔘 ICD-9-CM Code(s): _____)

44. Report 32

   🔘 CPT Code(s): _____

   🔘 ICD-10-CM Code(s): _____

   (🔘 ICD-9-CM Code(s): _____)

45. Report 33

   🔘 CPT Code(s): _____

   🔘 ICD-10-CM Code(s): _____

   (🔘 ICD-9-CM Code(s): _____)

46. Report 34

   🔘 CPT Code(s): _____

   🔘 ICD-10-CM Code(s): _____

   (🔘 ICD-9-CM Code(s): _____)

🔘 **User to decide number of codes necessary to correctly answer the question.**
Odd-numbered answers are located in Appendix B, while the full answer key is only available in the TEACH Instructor Resources on Evolve.

Copyright © 2016 by Elsevier Inc.

47. Report 35

    🔘 CPT Code(s): _____

    🔘 ICD-10-CM Code(s): _____

    (🔘 ICD-9-CM Code(s): _____)

48. Report 39

    🔘 CPT Code(s): _____

    🔘 ICD-10-CM Code(s): _____

    (🔘 ICD-9-CM Code(s): _____)

🔘 User to decide number of codes necessary to correctly answer the question.
Odd-numbered answers are located in Appendix B, while the full answer key is only available in the TEACH Instructor Resources on Evolve.

Copyright © 2016 by Elsevier Inc.

CHAPTER 20

Urinary and Male Genital Systems

THEORY

Make sure to check
evolve
for the latest
content updates

Urinary System Terminology

Without the use of reference material, match the following terms to the correct definitions:

1. _____ Calculus/calculi

2. _____ Cystolithectomy

3. _____ Cystometrogram (CMG)

4. _____ Endopyelotomy

5. _____ Exstrophy

6. _____ Nephrectomy

7. _____ Fulguration

8. _____ Kock pouch

9. _____ Lithotripsy

10. _____ Marsupialization

11. _____ Nephro-

12. _____ Nephrostomy

a. With the use of an endoscope, an incision is made to correct stenosis of the ureteropelvic junction

b. Kidney removal

c. Crushing of a gallbladder or urinary bladder stone followed by irrigation to wash the fragment out

d. A concretion of mineral salts, also called a stone

e. Surgical creation of a urinary bladder from a segment of the ileum

f. Condition in which an organ is turned inside out

g. Measurement of the pressures and capacity of the urinary bladder

h. Creation of a channel into the renal pelvis of the kidney

i. Surgical procedure that creates an open pouch from an internal abscess

j. Removal of a calculus from the urinary bladder

k. Use of electrical current to destroy tissue

l. Prefix meaning kidney

Odd-numbered answers are located in Appendix B, while the full answer key is only available in the TEACH Instructor Resources on Evolve.

Copyright © 2016 by Elsevier Inc.

Without the use of reference material, match the following terms to the correct definitions:

13. _____ Perivesical

14. _____ Perirenal

15. _____ Pyelo-

16. _____ Pyeloplasty

17. _____ Pyelostomy

18. _____ Renal pelvis

19. _____ Retroperitoneal

20. _____ Transureteroureterostomy

21. _____ Ureterolithotomy

22. _____ Ureterotomy

23. _____ Urethrocystography

24. _____ Urethrorrhaphy

a. Prefix meaning renal pelvis

b. Removal of a stone from the ureter

c. Surgical connection of one ureter to the other ureter

d. Surgical creation of an opening into the renal pelvis

e. Suturing of the urethra

f. Behind the sac holding the abdominal organs and viscera (peritoneum)

g. Around the kidney

h. Radiography of the bladder and urethra

i. Around the bladder

j. Funnel-shaped sac in the kidney where urine is received

k. Surgical reconstruction of the renal pelvis

l. Incision into the ureter

Male Genital Terminology

Without the use of reference material, match the following terms to the correct definitions:

25. _____ Cavernosa-saphenous

26. _____ Orchiectomy

27. _____ Hydrocele

28. _____ Vasogram

29. _____ Varicocele

30. _____ Vas deferens

a. Tube that carries sperm from the epididymis to the urethra

b. Swelling of a scrotal vein

c. Creation of a connection between the cavity of the penis and a vein

d. Castration

e. Sac of fluid

f. Recording of the flow in the vas deferens

Odd-numbered answers are located in Appendix B, while the full answer key is only available in the TEACH Instructor Resources on Evolve.

Copyright © 2016 by Elsevier Inc.

Without reference material, match the following terms to the correct definitions:

31. _____ Electrodesiccation

32. _____ Corpora cavernosa

33. _____ Epididymis

34. _____ Cavernosography

35. _____ Cavernosometry

36. _____ Plethysmography

37. _____ Hypospadias

38. _____ Vesiculectomy

39. _____ Prostatotomy

a. Excision of a seminal vesicle

b. Determining the changes in volume of an organ part or body

c. Incision into the prostate

d. Destruction of a lesion by the use of electrical current radiated through a needle

e. A tube located on the top of the testes that stores sperm

f. Measurements of the pressure in a cavity (e.g., penis)

g. Two cavities of the penis

h. Radiographic measurement of a cavity (e.g., the main part of the penis)

i. Congenital deformity of the urethra in which the urethral opening is on the underside of the penis rather than on the end

Without reference material, match the following terms to the correct definitions:

40. _____ Lymphadenectomy

41. _____ Priapism

42. _____ Chordee

43. _____ Urethroplasty

44. _____ Penoscrotal

45. _____ Spermatocele

a. Surgical repair of the urethra

b. Referring to the penis and scrotum

c. Painful condition in which the penis is constantly erect

d. Excision of lymph node(s)

e. Condition resulting in the penis being bent downward

f. Cyst filled with spermatozoa

Odd-numbered answers are located in Appendix B, while the full answer key is only available in the TEACH Instructor Resources on Evolve.

Copyright © 2016 by Elsevier Inc.

Without reference material, match the following terms to the correct definitions:

46. _____ Tumescence

47. _____ Cavernosa-corpus spongiosum shunt

48. _____ Cavernosa-glans penis fistulization

49. _____ Orchiopexy

50. _____ Vasovasostomy

51. _____ Vasovasorrhaphy

a. Creation of a connection between a cavity of the penis and the urethra

b. Creation of a connection between a cavity of the penis and the glans penis, which overlaps the penis cavity

c. Reversal of a vasectomy

d. Surgical procedure to release undescended testis

e. Suturing of the vas deferens

f. State of being swollen

Without reference material, match the following terms to the correct definitions:

52. _____ Epididymectomy

53. _____ Epididymovasostomy

54. _____ Vasotomy

55. _____ Vesiculotomy

56. _____ Seminal vesicle

57. _____ Tunica vaginalis

a. Creation of a new connection between the vas deferens and epididymis

b. Creation of an opening in the vas deferens

c. Covering of the testes

d. Incision into the seminal vesicle

e. Glands that secretes fluid that ultimately becomes semen

f. Surgical removal of the epididymis

Odd-numbered answers are located in Appendix B, while the full answer key is only available in the TEACH Instructor Resources on Evolve.

Copyright © 2016 by Elsevier Inc.

PRACTICAL

Using the CPT and ICD-10-CM/ICD-9-CM manuals, code the following:

58. Endoscopy for resection of primary malignant renal pelvis tumor through an established stoma.

    CPT Code:_____

    ICD-10-CM Code: _____

    (ICD-9-CM Code: _____)

59. Aspiration of a solitary, non-congenital renal cyst through percutaneous needle.

    CPT Code: _____

    ICD-10-CM Code: _____

    (ICD-9-CM Code: _____)

60. Ureteroureterostomy performed for urinary tract obstruction.

    CPT Code: _____

    ICD-10-CM Code: _____

    (ICD-9-CM Code: _____)

61. Transurethral incision of the prostate to treat benign hypertrophic prostatitis.

    CPT Code: _____

    ICD-10-CM Code: _____

    (ICD-9-CM Code: _____)

62. Cystourethroscopy due to intermittent hematuria.

    CPT Code: _____

    ICD-10-CM Code: _____

    (ICD-9-CM Code: _____)

63. Abdominal orchiopexy to release undescended intra-abdominal testes.

    CPT Code: _____

    ICD-10-CM Code: _____

    (ICD-9-CM Code: _____)

Odd-numbered answers are located in Appendix B, while the full answer key is only available in the TEACH Instructor Resources on Evolve.

Copyright © 2016 by Elsevier Inc.

64. Complicated prostatotomy of prostate cyst.

   CPT Code: _____

   ICD-10-CM Code: _____

   (ICD-9-CM Code: _____)

65. Closure of nephrocutaneous fistula.

   CPT Code: _____

66. A steroid injection for urethral stricture using a cystourethroscope.

   CPT Code(s): _____

67. Total urethrectomy of a 44-year-old male.

   CPT Code(s): _____

68. Circumcision using clamp, routine.

   CPT Code(s): _____

   ICD-10-CM Code(s): _____

   (ICD-9-CM Code(s): _____)

69. Excision of Skene's glands.

   CPT Code(s): _____

70. Bilateral shunt of corpora cavernosa–saphenous vein for priapism.

   CPT Code(s): _____

71. Vasovasorrhaphy.

   CPT Code(s): _____

72. Exposure of the prostate for insertion of radioactive substance.

   CPT Code(s): _____

73. Surgical reduction of torsion of testis with fixation of contralateral testis.

   CPT Code(s): _____

User to decide number of codes necessary to correctly answer the question.
Odd-numbered answers are located in Appendix B, while the full answer key is only available in the TEACH Instructor Resources on Evolve.

Copyright © 2016 by Elsevier Inc.

74. Distal hypospadias repair with chordee using a V-flap advancement, completed in one stage.

 CPT Code(s): _____

75. Simple destruction of four lesions of the penis using cryosurgery.

 CPT Code(s): _____

76. Repair of an incomplete circumcision.

 CPT Code(s): _____

77. Drainage of a scrotal wall abscess.

 CPT Code(s): _____

78. Ureterectomy, with repair of the bladder cuff.

 CPT Code(s): _____

 User to decide number of codes necessary to correctly answer the question.
Odd-numbered answers are located in Appendix B, while the full answer key is only available in the TEACH Instructor Resources on Evolve.

Copyright © 2016 by Elsevier Inc.

REPORTS

In Appendix A of this workbook you will find a section titled Reports, which contains original reports. Read the reports indicated below and supply the appropriate CPT and ICD-10-CM/ICD-9-CM codes on the following lines:

79. Report 36

    CPT Code(s): _____

80. Report 37

    CPT Code(s): _____

    ICD-10-CM Code(s): _____

    (ICD-9-CM Code(s): _____)

81. Report 38

    CPT Code(s): _____

    ICD-10-CM Code(s): _____

    (ICD-9-CM Code(s): _____)

82. Report 81

    CPT Code(s): _____

83. Report 82

    CPT Code(s): _____

84. Report 83

    CPT Code(s): _____

    ICD-10-CM Code(s): _____

    (ICD-9-CM Code(s): _____)

85. Report 84

    CPT Code(s): _____

 User to decide number of codes necessary to correctly answer the question.

Odd-numbered answers are located in Appendix B, while the full answer key is only available in the TEACH Instructor Resources on Evolve.

Copyright © 2016 by Elsevier Inc.

CHAPTER 21

Reproductive, Intersex Surgery, Female Genital System, and Maternity Care and Delivery

THEORY

Make sure to check
evolve
for the latest
content updates

Female Genital Terminology

Without the use of reference material, match the following terms to the correct definitions:

1. _____ Vulva

2. _____ Perineum

3. _____ Introitus

4. _____ Vagina

5. _____ Cervix uteri

6. _____ Corpus uteri

7. _____ Oviduct

8. _____ Salpingo-

9. _____ Oophor-

10. _____ Curettage

11. _____ Dilation

12. _____ Cystocele

13. _____ Rectocele

a. Herniation of the bladder into the vagina

b. Rounded, cone-shaped neck of the uterus, part of it protruding into the vagina

c. Prefix meaning ovary

d. External female genitalia, including labia majora, labia minora, clitoris, and vaginal opening

e. Uterus

f. Herniation of the rectal wall through the posterior wall of the vagina

g. Prefix meaning tube

h. Opening or entrance to the vagina

i. Scraping of a cavity using a spoon-shaped instrument

j. Expansion

k. Area between the vulva and anus

l. Canal from the external female genitalia to the uterus

m. Fallopian tube

Odd-numbered answers are located in Appendix B, while the full answer key is only available in the TEACH Instructor Resources on Evolve.

Reproductive, Intersex Surgery, Female Genital System, and Maternity Care and Delivery

Maternity Care and Delivery Terminology

Without the use of reference material, match the following terms to the correct definitions:

14. _____ Antepartum
15. _____ Postpartum
16. _____ Abortion
17. _____ Delivery
18. _____ Cesarean
19. _____ Ectopic
20. _____ Version
21. _____ Amniocentesis
22. _____ Cordocentesis
23. _____ Chorionic villus sampling (CVS)
24. _____ Hysterotomy
25. _____ Salpingectomy
26. _____ Oophorectomy
27. _____ Hysterectomy
28. _____ Hysterorrhaphy
29. _____ Tocolysis
30. _____ VBAC

a. Turning of the fetus from a presentation other than cephalic (head down) to cephalic for ease of birth
b. Termination of pregnancy
c. Surgical opening through abdominal wall for delivery
d. Before childbirth
e. After childbirth
f. Pregnancy outside the uterus (e.g., in the fallopian tube)
g. Childbirth
h. Incision into the uterus
i. Surgical removal of the uterus
j. Percutaneous aspiration of amniotic fluid
k. Surgical removal of ovary
l. Biopsy of the outermost part of the placenta
m. Suturing of the uterus
n. Repression of uterine contractions
o. Surgical removal of a fallopian tube
p. Vaginal delivery after previous cesarean delivery
q. Procedure to obtain a fetal blood sample, also called a percutaneous umbilical blood sampling

Odd-numbered answers are located in Appendix B, while the full answer key is only available in the TEACH Instructor Resources on Evolve.

Copyright © 2016 by Elsevier Inc.

Without the use of reference material, answer the following:

31. Plastic repair of the _____ is surgical repair of the opening to the vagina.

32. An incision into the vagina to gain access to the pelvic cavity is

    _____.

33. The insertion of a long needle into the back wall of the vagina to gain

    access to a peritoneal cul de sac abscess is _____.

34. A vaginal support device is a(n) _____.

35. When reporting the service of the introduction of a diaphragm, the cost of the diaphragm is included in the introduction.

    True or False? _____

36. The term that describes the procedure in which the surgeon strengthens the wall of the weakened vagina by pulling together the weakened vaginal area with sutures is:

    _____

37. The microscope that is used to view the vagina is a(n)

    _____.

38. The services described in the Manipulation category of the Vagina

    subheading require this type of anesthesia: _____

39. LEEP means _____.

40. Endometrial _____ is a biopsy of the mucous lining of the uterus.

41. What one procedure represents the majority of the codes in the Corpus

    Uteri subheading? _____

42. Hydatidiform mole, also known as a "molar pregnancy," results from genetic abnormalities.

    True or False? _____

43. A hysterosalpingography would have a component code from what

    section of the CPT manual? _____

Odd-numbered answers are located in Appendix B, while the full answer key is only available in the TEACH Instructor Resources on Evolve.

Copyright © 2016 by Elsevier Inc.

44. The first rule of a laparoscopy is that a surgical laparoscopy always

    includes this type of laparoscopy: _____

45. In what subheading would you find the codes to report fallopian tube services?

    _____

46. The three methods of tubal ligation are ligation, _____,

    and _____.

47. Gestation is divided into three time periods that are termed

    _____.

48. The first gestation time period is LMP to less than _____ weeks

    0 days, the second is _____ weeks 0 days to less than

    _____ weeks 0 days, and the third is _____ weeks 0 days
    until delivery.

49. What does EDD stand for?

    _____ _____ of _____

50. Preparation of the cervix for birth or dilation is termed cervical

    _____.

51. If a physician other than the attending provided only one office visit to
    a patient before delivery, a code from what section of the CPT manual

    would be used to report this service? _____

52. The time after delivery is referred to as _____.

Odd-numbered answers are located in Appendix B, while the full answer key is only available in the TEACH Instructor Resources on Evolve.

Copyright © 2016 by Elsevier Inc.

PRACTICAL

Using the CPT manual, code the following:

53. Dilation of the vagina under anesthesia.

    CPT Code: _____

54. Plastic repair of a urethrocele.

    CPT Code: _____

55. Labial adhesions lysis.

    CPT Code: _____

56. Simple complete vulvectomy.

    CPT Code: _____

57. Surgical hysteroscopy with polypectomy and dilatation and curettage.

    CPT Code: _____

58. Transposition of the left ovary.

    CPT Code: _____

59. Bilateral wedge resection of ovaries.

    CPT Code: _____

60. Therapeutic amniocentesis with amniotic fluid reduction.

    CPT Code: _____

61. Drainage of a cyst of the left ovary using the vaginal approach.

    CPT Code(s): _____

62. Surgical treatment of a second-trimester missed abortion.

    CPT Code(s): _____

63. Cesarean delivery only.

    CPT Code(s): _____

64. Hysterorrhaphy of a ruptured, pregnant uterus.

    CPT Code(s): _____

 User to decide number of codes necessary to correctly answer the question.
Odd-numbered answers are located in Appendix B, while the full answer key is only available in the TEACH Instructor Resources on Evolve.

65. Fetal contraction stress tests, antepartum.

🔾 CPT Code(s): _____

66. Radical vaginal hysterectomy.

🔾 CPT Code(s): _____

67. Marsupialization of Bartholin's gland cyst.

🔾 CPT Code(s): _____

68. Excision of Bartholin's gland.

🔾 CPT Code(s): _____

69. Destruction of extensive vaginal lesions.

🔾 CPT Code(s): _____

🔾 User to decide number of codes necessary to correctly answer the question.
Odd-numbered answers are located in Appendix B, while the full answer key is only available in the TEACH Instructor Resources on Evolve.

138

Copyright © 2016 by Elsevier Inc.

REPORTS

In Appendix A of this workbook you will find a section titled Reports, which contains original reports. Code only the primary surgery. Read the report indicated below and supply the appropriate CPT and ICD-10-CM/ICD-9-CM codes on the following lines:

70. Report 20

    ✿ CPT Code(s): _____

    ✿ ICD-10-CM Code(s): _____

    (✿ ICD-9-CM Code(s): _____)

71. Report 28

    ✿ CPT Code(s): _____

    ✿ ICD-10-CM Code(s): _____

    (✿ ICD-9-CM Code(s): _____)

72. Report 29

    ✿ CPT Code(s): _____

    ✿ ICD-10-CM Code(s): _____

    (✿ ICD-9-CM Code(s): _____)

73. Report 30

    ✿ CPT Code(s): _____

    ✿ ICD-10-CM Code(s): _____

    (✿ ICD-9-CM Code(s): _____)

✿ **User to decide number of codes necessary to correctly answer the question.**
Odd-numbered answers are located in Appendix B, while the full answer key is only available in the TEACH Instructor Resources on Evolve.

CHAPTER 22

Endocrine and Nervous Systems

THEORY

Endocrine System Terminology

Match the following terms to the correct definitions:

1. _____ Isthmus

2. _____ Isthmus, thyroid

3. _____ Isthmusectomy

4. _____ Contralateral

5. _____ Thyroidectomy

6. _____ Thyroglossal duct

7. _____ Thymectomy

8. _____ Adrenal

9. _____ Thyroid

10. _____ Thymus

11. _____ Parathyroid

a. Glands located on the top of the kidneys that produce steroid hormones

b. Produces a hormone to mobilize calcium from the bones to the blood

c. Connection of two regions or structures

d. Surgical removal of the thyroid

e. Produces hormones important to the immune response

f. Surgical removal of the isthmus

g. Surgical removal of the thymus

h. Part of the endocrine system, a gland that produces hormones that regulate metabolism

i. Tissue connection between right and left thyroid lobes

j. Develops in the embryo stage after the formation of the thyroid gland

k. Affecting the opposite side

Odd-numbered answers are located in Appendix B, while the full answer key is only available in the TEACH Instructor Resources on Evolve.

Copyright © 2016 by Elsevier Inc.

Nervous System Terminology

Match the following terms to the correct definitions:

12. _____ Cranium

13. _____ Skull

14. _____ Stereotaxis

15. _____ Laminectomy

16. _____ Somatic nerve

17. _____ Sympathetic nerve

18. _____ Peripheral nerves

19. _____ Shunt

20. _____ Central Nervous System

a. A method of identifying a specific area or point in the brain

b. Part of the peripheral nervous system that controls automatic body function; activated under stress

c. That part of the skeleton that encloses the brain

d. Divert or make an artificial passage

e. Twelve pairs of cranial nerves, 31 pairs of spinal nerves, and autonomic nervous system; connects peripheral receptors to the brain and spinal cord

f. Sensory or motor nerve

g. Entire skeletal framework of the head

h. Surgical excision of the lamina

i. Brain and spinal cord

Odd-numbered answers are located in Appendix B, while the full answer key is only available in the TEACH Instructor Resources on Evolve.

Copyright © 2016 by Elsevier Inc.

PRACTICAL

Using the CPT manual, code the following:

21. Incision and drainage of an infected thyroglossal duct cyst.

    ✧ CPT Code(s): _____

22. Removal of a complete cerebrospinal fluid shunt system; without replacement.

    ✧ CPT Code(s): _____

23. Suture of the posterior tibial nerve.

    ✧ CPT Code(s): _____

24. Lumbar sympathetic block (left).

    CPT Code: _____

25. Microdissection, microrepair ulnar digital nerve left middle finger.

    CPT Codes: _____, _____

26. Placement of a dorsal column stimulator with implanted generator, with stereotactic stimulation of spinal cord.

    CPT Code: _____

27. Epidural injection of a steroid, caudal.

    CPT Code: _____

28. Craniotomy for drainage of an intracranial abscess; infratentorial.

    CPT Code: _____

29. Re-operation, skull base surgery, repair of dura mater due to leak of CSF of middle cranial fossa; myocutaneous flap graft.

    CPT Code: _____

30. Insertion of a cerebrospinal fluid ventriculoperitoneal shunt for hydrocephalus.

    CPT Code: _____

31. Hemilaminectomy, posterior approach, with decompression of two nerve roots and with excision of herniated disc at L1-L2 and foraminotomy at L2-L3.

    CPT Codes: _____, _____

✧ **User to decide number of codes necessary to correctly answer the question.**

Odd-numbered answers are located in Appendix B, while the full answer key is only available in the TEACH Instructor Resources on Evolve.

Copyright © 2016 by Elsevier Inc.

REPORTS

In Appendix A of this workbook you will find a section titled Reports, which contains original reports. Read the reports indicated below and supply the appropriate CPT and ICD-10-CM/ICD-9-CM codes on the following lines:

32. Report 41

    CPT Codes: _____ (arthrodesis with discectomy),

    _____ (arthrodesis with discectomy), _____

    (instrumentation), _____ (allograft),

    _____ (evoked potential)

    ICD-10-CM Code: _____

    (ICD-9-CM Code: _____)

33. Report 43

    🔵 Code(s): _____

    🔵 ICD-10-CM Code(s): _____

    (🔵 ICD-9-CM Code(s): _____)

🔵 **User to decide number of codes necessary to correctly answer the question.**
Odd-numbered answers are located in Appendix B, while the full answer key is only available in the TEACH Instructor Resources on Evolve.

 Copyright © 2016 by Elsevier Inc.

CHAPTER 23

Eye, Ocular Adnexa, Auditory, and Operating Microscope

THEORY

Eye and Ocular Adnexa Terminology

Match the following terms to the correct definitions:

1. _____ Keratoplasty
2. _____ Evisceration
3. _____ Enucleation
4. _____ Exenteration
5. _____ Cataract
6. _____ Sclera
7. _____ Conjunctiva
8. _____ Uveal
9. _____ Tarsorrhaphy
10. _____ Ocular adnexa

a. Surgical repair of the cornea

b. Removal of an eye

c. Opaque covering on or in the lens

d. Lining of the eyelids and covering of the sclera

e. Removal of an organ all in one piece

f. Pulling the viscera outside the body through an incision

g. White outer portion of the eyeball

h. Vascular tissue of the choroids, ciliary body, and iris

i. Suturing together of the eyelids

j. Orbit, extraocular muscles, and eyelid

Odd-numbered answers are located in Appendix B, while the full answer key is only available in the TEACH Instructor Resources on Evolve.

Match the following terms to the correct definitions:

11. _____ Anterior segment

12. _____ Posterior segment

13. _____ Blephar/o-

14. _____ Cor/o-

15. _____ Cyclo/o-

16. _____ Dacry/o-

17. _____ Kerat/o-

18. _____ Ocul/o-

19. _____ Dacryocyst/o-

20. _____ Vitre/o-

21. _____ Astigmatism

22. _____ Strabismus

a. Prefix meaning eye

b. Prefix meaning tear/tear duct

c. Parts of the eye located behind the lens

d. Prefix meaning cornea

e. Prefix meaning pertaining to the vitreous body of the eye

f. Prefix meaning ciliary body or eye muscle

g. Parts of the eye in the front of and including the lens, orbit, extraocular muscles, and eyelid

h. Prefix meaning pertaining to the lacrimal sac

i. Extraocular muscle deviation resulting in unequal visual axes

j. Condition in which the refractive surfaces of the eyes are unequal

k. Prefix meaning eyelid

l. Prefix meaning pupil

Odd-numbered answers are located in Appendix B, while the full answer key is only available in the TEACH Instructor Resources on Evolve.

Copyright © 2016 by Elsevier Inc.

Auditory System Terminology

Match the following terms to the correct definitions:

23. _____ Aural atresia

24. _____ Transmastoid antrostomy

25. _____ Labyrinth

26. _____ Tympanic neurectomy

27. _____ Fenestration

28. _____ Parts of the external ear

29. _____ Parts of the middle ear

30. _____ Parts of the inner ear

31. _____ Mastoid-

32. _____ Myring-

33. _____ Audi-

34. _____ Exostosis

35. _____ Oto-

36. _____ Salping(o)-

37. _____ Apicectomy

a. Prefix meaning hearing

b. Auricle, pinna, external acoustic, and meatus

c. Prefix meaning ear

d. Prefix meaning (eustachian) tube

e. Vestibule, semicircular canals, and cochlea

f. Excision of the tympanic nerve

g. Congenital absence of the external auditory canal

h. Creation of a new opening (e.g., on the inner wall of the middle ear)

i. Malleus, incus, and stapes

j. A bony growth

k. Prefix meaning posterior temporal bone

l. Excision of a portion of the temporal bone

m. Called a simple mastoidectomy, it creates an opening in the mastoid for drainage

n. Inner connecting cavities, such as the internal ear

o. Prefix meaning eardrum

Odd-numbered answers are located in Appendix B, while the full answer key is only available in the TEACH Instructor Resources on Evolve.

Copyright © 2016 by Elsevier Inc.

PRACTICAL

Using the CPT and ICD-10-CM/ICD-9-CM manuals, code the following:

38. Incision and drainage of conjunctival cysts of left and right eyes.

    🟤 CPT Code(s): _____

    🟤 ICD-10-CM Code(s): _____

    (🟤 ICD-9-CM Code(s): _____)

39. Optic nerve decompression of the right eye.

    🟤 CPT Code(s): _____

40. Removal of an embedded foreign body of the upper left eyelid.

    CPT Code: _____

    ICD-10-CM Code: _____

    (ICD-9-CM Code: _____)

41. Myringoplasty of the left ear.

    🟤 CPT Code(s): _____

42. Single stage reconstruction of the right external auditory canal for congenital atresia.

    CPT Code: _____

    ICD-10-CM Code: _____

    (ICD-9-CM Code: _____)

43. Left stapedectomy with footplate drill out.

    🟤 CPT Code(s): _____

44. Excision of a lacrimal sac, left eye.

    🟤 CPT Code(s): _____

🟤 **User to decide number of codes necessary to correctly answer the question.**
Odd-numbered answers are located in Appendix B, while the full answer key is only available in the TEACH Instructor Resources on Evolve.

Copyright © 2016 by Elsevier Inc.

REPORTS

In Appendix A of this workbook you will find a section titled Reports, which contains original reports. Read the reports indicated below and supply the appropriate CPT and ICD-10-CM/ICD-9-CM codes on the following lines:

45. Report 85

    CPT Code: _____

    ICD-10-CM Code: _____

    (ICD-9-CM Codes: _____, _____)

46. Report 86

    🔵 CPT Code(s): _____

47. Report 87

    🔵 CPT Code(s): _____

48. Report 88

    🔵 CPT Code(s): _____

🔵 **User to decide number of codes necessary to correctly answer the question.**
Odd-numbered answers are located in Appendix B, while the full answer key is only available in the TEACH Instructor Resources on Evolve.

Copyright © 2016 by Elsevier Inc.

CHAPTER 24

Radiology

THEORY

Make sure to check **evolve** for the latest content updates

Match the following terms to the correct definitions:

1. _____ Anterior (ventral)

2. _____ Posterior (dorsal)

3. _____ Superior

4. _____ Inferior

5. _____ Medial

6. _____ Lateral

a. Toward the midline of the body

b. Toward the head or the upper part of the body; also known as cephalad or cephalic

c. In front of

d. Away from the midline of the body (to the side)

e. In back of

f. Away from the head or the lower part of the body; also known as caudad or caudal

Match the following radiographic procedures to the correct structures imaged:

7. _____ Fluoroscopy

8. _____ Magnetic resonance imaging (MRI)

9. _____ Tomography

10. _____ Xeroradiography

11. _____ Barium

12. _____ Biometry

a. Radiographic contrast medium

b. Procedure for viewing the interior of the body using x-rays and projecting the image onto a television screen

c. Photoelectric process of radiographs

d. Application of a statistical method to a biological fact

e. Procedure that uses nonionizing radiation to view the body in a cross-sectional view

f. Procedure that allows viewing of a single plane of the body by blurring out all but that particular level

Odd-numbered answers are located in Appendix B, while the full answer key is only available in the TEACH Instructor Resources on Evolve.

Copyright © 2016 by Elsevier Inc.

Match the following radiographic procedures to the correct structures imaged:

13. _____ Arthrography

14. _____ Cholangiography

15. _____ Cystography

16. _____ Discography

17. _____ Epididymography

18. _____ Hysterosalpingography

19. _____ Lymphangiography

20. _____ Myelography

21. _____ Urography

22. _____ Venography

a. Uterine cavity and fallopian tubes

b. Intervertebral joint

c. Kidneys, renal pelvis, ureters, and bladder

d. Bile ducts

e. Joint

f. Veins and tributaries

g. Subarachnoid space of the spine

h. Epididymis

i. Urinary bladder

j. Lymphatic vessels and nodes

Odd-numbered answers are located in Appendix B, while the full answer key is only available in the TEACH Instructor Resources on Evolve.

Copyright © 2016 by Elsevier Inc.

PRACTICAL

Using the CPT and ICD-10-CM/ICD-9-CM manuals, answer the following:

23. What is the unlisted diagnostic nuclear medicine code reported for cardiovascular procedures?

   CPT Code: _____

24. What is the add-on code for the coronary artery transcatheter placement during coronary intravascular brachytherapy for delivery of the radiation device?

   Code: _____

25. The modifier to indicate only the professional component was provided.

   Modifier: _____

26. The modifier to indicate only the technical component was provided.

   Modifier: _____

27. Supervision and interpretation of angiography, spinal artery, selective. Report radiology service only.

   CPT Code: _____

28. Radiological examination of the eye for foreign body.

   CPT Code: _____

29. Radiological examination of mastoids, four views per side.

   CPT Code: _____

30. Radiological examination of the ribs, unilateral, two views.

   CPT Code: _____

31. MRI of the neck, with contrast material.

   CPT Code: _____

32. Computed tomography of the thoracic spine, without contrast.

   CPT Code: _____

33. Hip x-ray study, unilateral, two views.

   CPT Code: _____

Odd-numbered answers are located in Appendix B, while the full answer key is only available in the TEACH Instructor Resources on Evolve.

34. Complete four-view radiological examination of the wrist.

    CPT Code: _____

35. Radiological examination of a surgical specimen.

    CPT Code: _____

36. An established patient is seen in the clinic office complaining of severe headaches. To diagnose and treat the patient, the physician needs to identify a cause for these headaches. He performs an expanded problem focused history and examination and orders a CT scan of the head. The clinic radiologist performed the x-ray in which contrast was used.

    CPT Codes: _____ (physician), _____ (radiologist)

37. A new patient is admitted to the hospital on an observation status after a fall at home. A comprehensive history is collected and a general, multisystem comprehensive physical examination is performed. After talking to the patient and relatives and performing the examination, the physician finds that the patient has a number of symptoms that are usually due to an increase in intracranial pressure. The physician considers this patient's problems to be of moderately severe complexity. The MDM complexity is moderate. A CT scan of the brain without contrast is done. Brain lesions are discovered, and the physician advises radiation therapy. The patient is sent to the clinic's radiology department, where an A-scan bilateral ophthalmic biometry by ultrasound is done. The patient later has therapeutic radiology treatment planning that is simple. Later the patient has radiation treatment delivery to a single area up to 5 MeV. The patient continues with weekly radiology therapy management, five treatments.

    CPT Codes: _____, _____,

    _____, _____, _____,

    _____

38. A new patient is seen in the clinic for an office consult. The patient has a mass in the neck with related pain and dysphagia. The consulting physician performs an expanded problem focused history and examination, and low-complexity decision making. A CT scan of the patient's neck is ordered. This was done with and without contrast.

    ☕ CPT Code(s): _____

☕ User to decide number of codes necessary to correctly answer the question.

Odd-numbered answers are located in Appendix B, while the full answer key is only available in the TEACH Instructor Resources on Evolve.

Copyright © 2016 by Elsevier Inc.

39. A patient was admitted to the hospital for removal of a pericardial clot. The physician orders a real-time chest ultrasound. Chest magnetic resonance (proton) imaging is also ordered (without contrast). A pericardiotomy is performed for removal of clot.

    CPT Code(s): _____

40. Radiological examination, ankle, two views.

    CPT Code(s): _____

41. X-ray of a 6-month-old's upper arm; 2 views.

    CPT Code(s): _____

42. Unilateral selective pulmonary angiography, supervision and interpretation. Report radiology service only.

    CPT Code(s): _____

43. Fluoroscopic guidance for needle placement.

    CPT Code(s): _____

44. Computed tomography guidance for stereotactic localization.

    CPT Code(s): _____

45. Transrectal ultrasound.

    CPT Code(s): _____

46. Four-view x-ray of the lumbosacral spine.

    CPT Code(s): _____

47. Myelography, cervical, radiological supervision and interpretation.

    CPT Code(s): _____

48. Bilateral screening mammography.

    CPT Code(s): _____

49. X-ray of the facial bones, 2 views.

    CPT Code(s): _____

50. TMJ x-ray with mouth open and closed on one side of the mouth.

    CPT Code(s): _____

 User to decide number of codes necessary to correctly answer the question.

Odd-numbered answers are located in Appendix B, while the full answer key is only available in the TEACH Instructor Resources on Evolve.

Copyright © 2016 by Elsevier Inc.

51. X-ray of abdomen, single anteroposterior, and additional oblique and cone views.

    ⊛ CPT Code(s): _____

52. Placement of a long gastrointestinal tube, including fluoroscopy, radiological supervision and interpretation. Report radiology service only.

    ⊛ CPT Code(s): _____

53. Venography, superior sagittal sinus, radiological supervision and interpretation for thrombosis of intracranial venous sinus. Report radiology service only.

    CPT Code: _____

    ICD-10-CM Code: _____

    (ICD-9-CM Code: _____)

54. Magnetic resonance spectroscopy for temporal meningioma, benign.

    CPT Code: _____

    ICD-10-CM Code: _____

    (ICD-9-CM Code: _____)

55. Intravascular ultrasound of a noncoronary vessel, radiological supervision and interpretation due to renal artery stenosis.

    CPT Code: _____

    ICD-10-CM Code: _____

    (ICD-9-CM Code: _____)

56. Venography of unilateral extremity; radiological supervision and interpretation in a patient with end-stage renal disease on hemodialysis. Report radiology service only.

    CPT Code: _____

    ICD-10-CM Codes: _____, _____

    (ICD-9-CM Codes: _____, _____)

⊛ User to decide number of codes necessary to correctly answer the question.

Odd-numbered answers are located in Appendix B, while the full answer key is only available in the TEACH Instructor Resources on Evolve.

Copyright © 2016 by Elsevier Inc.

REPORTS

In Appendix A of this workbook you will find a section titled Reports, which contains original reports. Read the reports indicated below and supply the appropriate CPT and ICD-10-CM/ICD-9-CM codes on the following lines:

57. Report 45

    CPT Code: _____

    ICD-10-CM Code: _____

    (ICD-9-CM Code: _____)

58. Report 46

    CPT Code: _____

    ICD-10-CM Code: _____

    (ICD-9-CM Code: _____)

59. Report 47

    CPT Code: _____

    ICD-10-CM Code: _____

    (ICD-9-CM Code: _____)

60. Report 48

    CPT Code: _____

    ICD-10-CM Code: _____

    (ICD-9-CM Code: _____)

61. Report 49

    CPT Code(s): _____

    ICD-10-CM Code(s): _____

    (ICD-9-CM Code(s): _____)

62. Report 50

User to decide number of codes necessary to correctly answer the question.
Odd-numbered answers are located in Appendix B, while the full answer key is only available in the TEACH Instructor Resources on Evolve.

🌀 CPT Code(s): _____

🌀 ICD-10-CM Code(s): _____

(🌀 ICD-9-CM Code(s): _____)

63. Report 51

🌀 CPT Code(s): _____

🌀 ICD-10-CM Code(s): _____

(🌀 ICD-9-CM Code(s): _____)

64. Report 52

🌀 CPT Code(s): _____

🌀 ICD-10-CM Code(s): _____

(🌀 ICD-9-CM Code(s): _____)

65. Report 53

🌀 CPT Code(s): _____

🌀 ICD-10-CM Code(s): _____

(🌀 ICD-9-CM Code(s): _____)

🌀 **User to decide number of codes necessary to correctly answer the question.**
Odd-numbered answers are located in Appendix B, while the full answer key is only available in the TEACH Instructor Resources on Evolve.

Copyright © 2016 by Elsevier Inc.

CHAPTER 25

Pathology/Laboratory

THEORY

Make sure to check
evolve
for the latest
content updates

Without the use of reference materials, answer the following:

1. In what section of the CPT manual will you find the codes to indicate

   the service of venipuncture? _____

2. When a laboratory drug test is qualitative, it measures the

   _____ of the drug.

3. When a laboratory drug test is quantitative, it measures the

   _____ and the _____ of a specific drug.

4. When coding an evocative/suppression test, you may have an E/M code
   to indicate a prolonged period of time the physician spends with the
   patient during the testing process or a report of the injection or
   infusion service. What other service may you need to report?

   _____

5. A sample of tissue from a suspect area that is examined by a pathologist
   is a specimen, a block is a frozen piece of the specimen, and a(n)

   _____ is a slice of the frozen block.

6. How many levels of surgical pathology are there? _____

7. If one breast specimen is received for pathological analysis and the
   pathologist examines two blocks of the specimen, how many codes

   would be used to report the service of analysis? _____

**Odd-numbered answers are located in Appendix B, while the full answer key is only available in the TEACH
Instructor Resources on Evolve.**

Copyright © 2016 by Elsevier Inc.

PRACTICAL

Using the CPT and ICD-10-CM/ICD-9-CM manuals, code the following:

8. CARDIAC ENZYMES in a patient newly diagnosed with an acute inferior myocardial infarction.

Ref	Range	Units	12/18/XX
CPK	35-232 IU	69	0.0123
CKMB	0-10	ng/ml	1

CARDIAC MARKERS
12/18/XX   +123 TROPONIN I   <0.3 ng/ml

Troponin I Interpretation

≤0.4 ng/ml for apparently healthy individual

0.5-1.9 ng/ml for clinically Dx non-AMI patients

≥2.0 g/ml reasonably specific for AMI

CPT Codes: CPK, total: _____

CKMB (creatine kinase, cardiac fraction):

_____

Troponin, quantitative: _____

ICD-10-CM Code: _____

(ICD-9-CM Code: _____)

9. GENERAL BLOOD CHEMISTRY in a patient with dehydration, joint pains, and fever.

Ref	Range	Units	10/30/XX 0620	10/27/XX 1855
BUN	7-22	mg/dl		H 37
Sodium	136-145	mmol/L		138
Potassium	3.6-5.5	mmol/L		4.5
Creatinine	0.6-1.3	mg/dl	H 1.9	H 2.4
Uric acid	2.6-6.0	mg/dl	H 9.6	

CPT Codes: BUN: _____

Sodium: _____

Potassium: _____

Creatinine: _____

Uric acid: _____

Odd-numbered answers are located in Appendix B, while the full answer key is only available in the TEACH Instructor Resources on Evolve.

Copyright © 2016 by Elsevier Inc.

ICD-10-CM Codes: _____, _____, _____

(ICD-9-CM Codes: _____, _____,

_____)

10. An 84-year-old monitored for diagnoses of renal failure, anemia, and hypertension.

CPT Codes: Labs include:

Magnesium: _____

Iron: _____

Phosphorus: _____

Total protein serum: _____

ICD-10-CM Codes: _____, _____, _____

(ICD-9-CM Codes: _____, _____,

_____)

11. A 48-year-old female patient with hyperlipidemia, currently on Lipitor.

CPT Codes: Labs include:

Hepatic function: _____

Lipid panel: _____

ICD-10-CM Code: _____

(ICD-9-CM Code: _____)

12. A 20-year-old male in for labs due to chronic asthma.

CPT Codes: Labs include:

Theophylline: _____

ICD-10-CM Code: _____

(ICD-9-CM Code: _____)

13. A 55-year-old male in for labs, total digoxin level for chronic atrial fibrillation.

CPT Codes: Labs include:

Digoxin; total: _____

ICD-10-CM Code:_____

(ICD-9-CM Code: _____)

Odd-numbered answers are located in Appendix B, while the full answer key is only available in the TEACH Instructor Resources on Evolve.

Copyright © 2016 by Elsevier Inc.

REPORTS

In Appendix A of this workbook you will find a section titled Reports, which contains original reports. Read the reports indicated below and supply the appropriate CPT and ICD-10-CM/ICD-9-CM codes on the following lines:

14. Report 54

    🖱 CPT Code(s): _____

    🖱 ICD-10-CM Code(s): _____

    (🖱 ICD-9-CM Code(s): _____)

15. Report 55

    🖱 CPT Code(s): _____

    🖱 ICD-10-CM Code(s): _____

    (🖱 ICD-9-CM Code(s): _____)

16. Report 56

    🖱 CPT Code(s): _____

    🖱 ICD-10-CM Code(s): _____

    (🖱 ICD-9-CM Code(s): _____)

17. Report 57

    🖱 CPT Code(s): _____

    🖱 ICD-10-CM Code(s): _____

    (🖱 ICD-9-CM Code(s): _____)

18. Report 58

    🖱 CPT Code(s): _____

    🖱 ICD-10-CM Code(s): _____

    (🖱 ICD-9-CM Code(s): _____)

🖱 **User to decide number of codes necessary to correctly answer the question.**
Odd-numbered answers are located in Appendix B, while the full answer key is only available in the TEACH Instructor Resources on Evolve.

Copyright © 2016 by Elsevier Inc.

19. Report 59

    🌐 CPT Code(s): _____

    🌐 ICD-10-CM Code(s): _____

    (🌐 ICD-9-CM Code(s): _____)

20. Report 60

    🌐 CPT Code(s): _____

    🌐 ICD-10-CM Code(s): _____

    (🌐 ICD-9-CM Code(s): _____)

21. Report 61

    🌐 CPT Code(s): _____

    🌐 ICD-10-CM Code(s): _____

    (🌐 ICD-9-CM Code(s): _____)

22. Report 62

    🌐 CPT Code(s): _____

    🌐 ICD-10-CM Code(s): _____

    (🌐 ICD-9-CM Code(s): _____)

23. Report 63

    🌐 CPT Code(s): _____

    🌐 ICD-10-CM Code(s): _____

    (🌐 ICD-9-CM Code(s): _____)

24. Report 64

    🌐 CPT Code(s): _____

    🌐 ICD-10-CM Code(s): _____

    (🌐 ICD-9-CM Code(s): _____)

🌐 **User to decide number of codes necessary to correctly answer the question.**
Odd-numbered answers are located in Appendix B, while the full answer key is only available in the TEACH Instructor Resources on Evolve.

Copyright © 2016 by Elsevier Inc.

25. Report 65

    ⚛ CPT Code(s): _____

    ⚛ ICD-10-CM Code(s): _____

    (⚛ ICD-9-CM Code(s): _____)

26. Report 66

    ⚛ CPT Code(s): _____

    ⚛ ICD-10-CM Code(s): _____

    (⚛ ICD-9-CM Code(s): _____)

27. Report 67

    ⚛ CPT Code(s): _____

    ⚛ ICD-10-CM Code(s): _____

    (⚛ ICD-9-CM Code(s): _____)

⚛ User to decide number of codes necessary to correctly answer the question.

Odd-numbered answers are located in Appendix B, while the full answer key is only available in the TEACH Instructor Resources on Evolve.

Copyright © 2016 by Elsevier Inc.

CHAPTER 26

Medicine

THEORY

Without the use of reference material, match the following terms to the correct definitions:

1. _____ Aphakia
2. _____ Echography
3. _____ Gonioscopy
4. _____ Hemodialysis
5. _____ Modality
6. _____ Nystagmus
7. _____ Optokinetic
8. _____ Percutaneous
9. _____ Phlebotomy
10. _____ Retrograde
11. _____ Subcutaneous
12. _____ Tonometry
13. _____ Transcutaneous
14. _____ Tympanometry

a. Entering by way of the skin

b. Moving backward or against the usual direction of flow

c. Through the skin

d. Cleansing of the blood outside the body

e. Procedure for evaluation of middle ear disorders

f. Rapid involuntary eye movements

g. Cutting into a vein

h. Use of a scope to examine the angles of the eye

i. Movement of the eye to objects moving in the visual field

j. Ultrasound procedure in which sound waves are bounced off an internal organ and the resulting image is recorded

k. Measurement of pressure or tension

l. Tissue below dermis, primarily fat cells that insulate the body

m. Absence of the lens of the eye

n. Treatment method

Odd-numbered answers are located in Appendix B, while the full answer key is only available in the TEACH Instructor Resources on Evolve.

Copyright © 2016 by Elsevier Inc.

Match the following administration methods for drugs:

15. _____ OTH		a. Subcutaneous
16. _____ IT		b. Inhalant solution
17. _____ IV		c. Various routes
18. _____ IM		d. Intrathecal
19. _____ SC		e. Intramuscular
20. _____ INH		f. Intravenous
21. _____ VAR		g. Other routes

Define the following terms:

22. Oscillating _____

23. Audiometry _____

24. Tympanometry _____

25. Electrocochleography _____

26. Orthoptic _____

27. Angioscopy _____

28. Electroretinography _____

29. Anomaloscope _____

30. Aphakia _____

31. Corneosclera _____

32. Cornea _____

33. Sclera _____

Odd-numbered answers are located in Appendix B, while the full answer key is only available in the TEACH Instructor Resources on Evolve.

Copyright © 2016 by Elsevier Inc.

PRACTICAL

Using the CPT and ICD-10-CM/ICD-9-CM manuals, code the following:

34. Three injections of allergen with the provision of the extract and professional service.

    CPT Code: _____

35. Two photo patch tests.

    CPT Code: _____ × _____

36. Replacement of contact lenses.

    CPT Code: _____

37. Patient is fitted for bifocal spectacles.

    CPT Code: _____

38. Electro-oculography with interpretation and report.

    CPT Code: _____

39. Optokinetic nystagmus test.

    CPT Code: _____

40. Positional nystagmus test, with recording, five positions.

    CPT Code: _____

41. An esophagus acid reflux test with nasal catheter electrode placement for detection of gastroesophageal reflux.

    CPT Code: _____

42. Peritoneal dialysis with two (repeated) physician evaluations.

    CPT Code: _____

43. Hypnotherapy.

    CPT Code: _____

44. Bernstein test for esophagitis.

    CPT Code: _____

45. Evaluation of auditory rehabilitation status, 1 hour.

    CPT Code: _____

Odd-numbered answers are located in Appendix B, while the full answer key is only available in the TEACH Instructor Resources on Evolve.

46. Family psychotherapy without the patient present.

    CPT Code: _____

47. Hemodialysis access flow study to determine blood flow in grafts.

    CPT Code: _____

48. Puretone audiometry; air and bone.

    CPT Code: _____

49. Insertion of a Swan-Ganz catheter.

    CPT Code: _____

50. Electronic analysis for sick sinus syndrome of a single-chamber implantable defibrillator, with reprogramming (in person).

    CPT Code: _____

    ICD-10-CM Code: _____

    (ICD-9-CM Code: _____)

51. Ventilation management for assist of breathing; second day for a hospital inpatient. The patient has a diagnosis of acute respiratory failure.

    CPT Code: _____

    ICD-10-CM Code: _____

    (ICD-9-CM Code: _____)

52. Training for a prosthetic arm, 45 minutes.

    CPT Code(s): _____

53. Conscious sedation provided by the same physician performing the diagnostic test on a 40-year-old patient for 30 minutes.

    CPT Code(s): _____

54. GI tract intraluminal imaging from the esophagus through the ileum, with interpretation and report.

    CPT Code(s): _____

55. Administration of two vaccines.

    CPT Code(s): _____

User to decide number of codes necessary to correctly answer the question.

Odd-numbered answers are located in Appendix B, while the full answer key is only available in the TEACH Instructor Resources on Evolve.

Copyright © 2016 by Elsevier Inc.

56. The patient is being treated for bacterial endocarditis, on IV antibiotic therapy. The patient also has a new onset of ventricular flutter. The cardiologist documents a detailed history, detailed examination, and high medical decision making during this subsequent inpatient encounter.

  🔵 CPT Code(s): _____

  🔵 ICD-10-CM Code(s): _____

  (🔵 ICD-9-CM Code(s): _____)

57. The service provided to the patient was an initial episode of care for an acquired atrial septal defect due to acute myocardial infarction of the inferolateral wall. The patient was admitted to the hospital for care.

  ICD-10-CM Codes: _____, _____

  (ICD-9-CM Codes: _____, _____)

58. Arteriosclerosis of legs with intermittent claudication.

  ICD-10-CM Code: _____

  (ICD-9-CM Code: _____)

🔵 User to decide number of codes necessary to correctly answer the question.
Odd-numbered answers are located in Appendix B, while the full answer key is only available in the TEACH Instructor Resources on Evolve.

REPORTS

In Appendix A of this workbook you will find a section titled Reports, which contains original reports. Read the reports indicated below and supply the appropriate CPT and ICD-10-CM/ICD-9-CM codes on the following lines:

59. Report 68

    🔘 CPT Code(s): _____

    🔘 ICD-10-CM Code(s): _____

    (🔘 ICD-9-CM Code(s): _____)

60. Report 69

    🔘 CPT Code(s): _____

    🔘 ICD-10-CM Code(s): _____

    (🔘 ICD-9-CM Code(s): _____)

61. Report 70

    🔘 CPT Code(s): _____

62. Report 71

    🔘 CPT Code(s): _____

63. Report 72

    🔘 CPT Code(s): _____

64. Report 73

    🔘 CPT Code(s): _____

65. Report 74

    🔘 CPT Code(s): _____

    🔘 ICD-10-CM Code(s): _____

    (🔘 ICD-9-CM Code(s): _____)

66. Report 75

    🔘 CPT Code(s): _____

🔘 **User to decide number of codes necessary to correctly answer the question.**
Odd-numbered answers are located in Appendix B, while the full answer key is only available in the TEACH Instructor Resources on Evolve.

Copyright © 2016 by Elsevier Inc.

67. Report 76

    🜂 CPT Code(s): _____

    🜂 ICD-10-CM Code(s): _____

    (🜂 ICD-9-CM Code(s): _____)

68. Report 77

    🜂 CPT Code(s): _____

69. Report 78

    🜂 CPT Code(s): _____

    🜂 ICD-10-CM Code(s): _____

    (🜂 ICD-9-CM Code(s): _____)

70. Report 79

    🜂 CPT Code(s): _____

    🜂 ICD-10-CM Code(s): _____

    (🜂 ICD-9-CM Code(s): _____)

71. Report 80

    🜂 CPT Code(s): _____

🜂 **User to decide number of codes necessary to correctly answer the question.**
Odd-numbered answers are located in Appendix B, while the full answer key is only available in the TEACH Instructor Resources on Evolve.

Copyright © 2016 by Elsevier Inc.

CHAPTER 27

Inpatient Coding

THEORY

Without the use of reference material, complete the following:

1. In which setting would an ICD-10-PCS/ICD-9-CM procedure code be assigned for a herniorrhaphy?

   Inpatient   Outpatient

2. In which setting would documentation in the discharge summary of a suspected condition be coded as if it exists?

   Inpatient   Outpatient

3. In which setting would a CPT code be assigned for a cataract extraction?

   Inpatient   Outpatient

4. A significant procedure must be performed in an operating room.

   True   False

5. The use of a POA indicator is optional.

   True   False

6. If a patient is admitted from outpatient surgery for a complication, the reason for the surgery is the principal diagnosis.

   True   False

7. When two or more diagnoses equally meet the definition for principal diagnosis, the one that the physician lists first should be assigned as the principal diagnosis.

   True   False

Odd-numbered answers are located in Appendix B, while the full answer key is only available in the TEACH Instructor Resources on Evolve.

Copyright © 2016 by Elsevier Inc.

8. A patient is admitted with syncope. The physician documents that the patient's syncope is due to orthostatic hypotension or bradycardia. Which diagnosis(es) should be reported?
   a. syncope
   b. syncope, orthostatic hypotension, bradycardia
   c. orthostatic hypotension, bradycardia
   d. bradycardia

9. Patient is admitted with right lower quadrant pain and anorexia due to acute appendicitis. Which diagnosis(es) should be reported?
   a. acute appendicitis
   b. right lower quadrant pain, appendicitis
   c. acute appendicitis, anorexia, right lower quadrant pain
   d. anorexia, acute appendicitis

10. If it is documented that the patient has a low magnesium level and magnesium supplements are ordered, the coder should:
    a. query the physician regarding the significance of the abnormal lab value and subsequent treatment
    b. add a code for abnormal lab value
    c. check with supervisor
    d. all of the above

Using Table 32-1 located in the main textbook, answer the following:

11. Altering the route of passage of the contents of a tubular body part is:
    a. alteration
    b. bypass
    c. change device in
    d. control postprocedural bleeding in

12. Cutting into a body part without draining fluids and/or gases from the body part in order to separate or transect a body part is:
    a. alteration
    b. detachment
    c. division
    d. change device in

13. Physical eradication of all or a portion of a body part by the direct use of energy, force, or a destructive agent is:
    a. division
    b. excision
    c. destruction
    d. resection

14. An example of fragmentation is:
    a. lithotripsy
    b. spinal fusion
    c. dermabrasion
    d. cutdown

Odd-numbered answers are located in Appendix B, while the full answer key is only available in the TEACH Instructor Resources on Evolve.

Copyright © 2016 by Elsevier Inc.

15. An example of an occlusion type of procedure is:
    a. clamping
    b. clipping
    c. ligation
    d. all of the above

Odd-numbered answers are located in Appendix B, while the full answer key is only available in the TEACH Instructor Resources on Evolve.

SEQUENCING EXERCISES

Cases of Principal Diagnosis and Other Diagnoses

In the following cases, identify the principal diagnosis and other diagnoses using the ICD-10-CM Official Guidelines for Coding and Reporting. *This is a sequencing exercise, not a coding exercise. If there is only one diagnosis, write "none" for Other Diagnoses.*

16. Mr. Jones presents to the emergency department with complaints of leg pain, inflammation and swelling of the ankle and calf, and a fever. The day before he had been seen in the physician's office for treatment of cellulitis and was given antibiotics. Mr. Jones was admitted to the hospital for IV antibiotics.

    Principal Diagnosis: _____

    Other Diagnoses: _____

17. Mrs. Beatty was seen in her physician's office with a complaint of shortness of breath and chest pain. Dr. Adams admitted her with a diagnosis of congestive heart failure.

    Principal Diagnosis: _____

    Other Diagnoses: _____

18. Mr. Janes was admitted for colon resection for colon cancer and also had chemotherapy following surgery. Mr. Janes complained of joint pain while in the hospital, and an MRI showed metastases to bone.

    Principal Diagnosis: _____

    Other Diagnoses: _____

19. Mrs. Anderson had a hysterectomy and bilateral oophorectomy for ovarian cancer 1 week ago. It is planned that the patient will undergo chemotherapy. The patient is now admitted with internal hemorrhaging from the surgery site.

    Principal Diagnosis: _____

    Other Diagnoses: _____

20. Miss Nelson is admitted for a D&C for menorrhagia. During her preoperative physical examination, the physician notices she has a fever and her lungs are congested. He cancels surgery because the patient shows symptoms of acute bronchitis.

    Principal Diagnosis: _____

    Other Diagnoses: _____

Odd-numbered answers are located in Appendix B, while the full answer key is only available in the TEACH Instructor Resources on Evolve.

Copyright © 2016 by Elsevier Inc.

21. Jackie Jones was cooking at home and spilled a pot of boiling water on her arms, legs, and stomach. She presented to the emergency department with second-degree burns of the thighs and third-degree burns of the arms and stomach. She was admitted and taken directly to surgery.

    Principal Diagnosis: _____

    Other Diagnoses: _____

22. Mr. Anderson regularly sees a physician and is on medication for management of his chronic bronchitis. Last night he was complaining of coughing and difficulty breathing. He was admitted with a diagnosis of chronic bronchitis with acute exacerbation.

    Principal Diagnosis: _____

    Other Diagnoses: _____

23. Mrs. Smith is at 32 weeks' gestation and complaining of stomach cramps and diarrhea × 36 hours. She is admitted for rehydration with IV fluids and is diagnosed with dehydration and gastroenteritis. Pregnancy is felt to be incidental.

    Principal Diagnosis: _____

    Other Diagnoses: _____

Odd-numbered answers are located in Appendix B, while the full answer key is only available in the TEACH Instructor Resources on Evolve.

Copyright © 2016 by Elsevier Inc.

177

PRINCIPAL DIAGNOSIS

Provide the principal diagnosis code, the procedure code, and any additional diagnosis codes for the following:

24. **HISTORY OF PRESENT ILLNESS:** The patient is a 52-year-old male who was involved in an interpersonal altercation at approximately 1:30 in the morning. He presented to the emergency department with complaints of pain and swelling to the right side of the face. The patient had been struck multiple times with the butt end of a handgun. He denied loss of consciousness. The attack was witnessed, and the witnesses also claimed there was no loss of consciousness. He presented with pain and swelling on the right side of his face in the temporal region and in the right eye region. He had a small abrasion on the top of his head and on the right forehead. No lacerations were noted. He had no diplopia. The past medical history and past surgical history were noncontributory. The patient was taking no medications and had no allergies.

    HOSPITAL COURSE: Admission x-rays and CT scan revealed a nondisplaced right zygoma fracture and an orbital floor fracture with slight limitation on physical examination of his upward gaze. He was taken to the operating room for exploration and placement of a Silastic implant to the right orbital floor fracture, which was accomplished without difficulty and without complication. The patient tolerated the procedure well. Postoperative course was uncomplicated. He received IV antibiotics throughout his stay in the hospital.

    FINAL DIAGNOSIS: Right orbital fracture; right zygoma fracture; abrasion of head.

    ICD-10-CM PRINCIPAL DIAGNOSIS and CODE: _____

    ICD-10-CM OTHER DIAGNOSES and CODES:

    _____, _____, _____,

    _____

    ICD-10-PCS PROCEDURE CODE: _____

    ICD-9-CM PRINCIPAL DIAGNOSIS and CODE:

    _____

    ICD-9-CM OTHER DIAGNOSES and CODES: _____,

    _____, _____

    ICD-9-CM PROCEDURE CODE: _____

Odd-numbered answers are located in Appendix B, while the full answer key is only available in the TEACH Instructor Resources on Evolve.

Copyright © 2016 by Elsevier Inc.

25. **HISTORY OF PRESENT ILLNESS:** The patient is a 69-year-old, right-handed male who presents with a 4-day history of severe right-sided headache, visual blurring, and diplopia. The patient was seen in the ENT clinic for discharge from his right ear of 2 days' duration, diagnosed to be otitis externa on the day of admission. The patient was subsequently transferred from the clinic to the emergency department. The patient denied a history of seizure, motor or sensory deficit, nausea or vomiting, trauma, or speech difficulties. Past medical history of sinusitis for many years. Current medications are none. Allergies, none.

PHYSICAL EXAMINATION: HEENT: Right pupil 3 mm, nonreactive. Left pupil 2 mm, reactive. Disconjugate gaze present. Right ptosis. Oropharynx clear without lesions. The neck is supple without lymphadenopathy or thyromegaly. Heart: regular rate and rhythm without murmurs or gallops. Lungs clear to percussion and auscultation. The neurological examination: awake, alert, oriented times three, follows three simple commands. Cranial nerves, partial right third nerve palsy with ptosis, 3-mm nonreactive right pupil, right medial gaze with disconjugate extraocular eye movement. Motor is 5/5 throughout without drift. Finger test is within normal limits. The sensory is intact to fine touch and proprioception: cerebral examination within normal limits.

HOSPITAL COURSE: Patient was admitted with suspicion of intracranial aneurysm. On the following day, the patient underwent a three-vessel cerebral angiogram that demonstrated a posterior communicating artery aneurysm and questionable anterior communicating artery aneurysm. The patient underwent a right craniotomy for clipping of right posterior communicating artery aneurysm and anterior communicating artery aneurysm. Postoperatively, the patient was observed in the surgical intensive care unit until his mental status was stabilized. The palsy and ptosis noted preoperatively resolved during the postsurgical course. The patient has been ambulating without assistance and tolerating food well. The patient was also seen by the ENT service during the hospitalization for his otitis externa and their recommendations were followed.

FINAL DIAGNOSES: Right posterior communicating artery aneurysm; anterior communicating artery aneurysm; right otitis externa.

ICD-10-CM PRINCIPAL DIAGNOSIS and CODE: _____

ICD-10-CM OTHER DIAGNOSIS and CODE: _____

ICD-10-PCS PROCEDURE CODE: _____

ICD-9-CM PRINCIPAL DIAGNOSIS and CODE:

_____

ICD-9-CM OTHER DIAGNOSIS and CODE: _____

ICD-9-CM PROCEDURE CODE: _____

Odd-numbered answers are located in Appendix B, while the full answer key is only available in the TEACH Instructor Resources on Evolve.

Copyright © 2016 by Elsevier Inc.

Reports

> NOTE: These reports are meant to be referenced as exercises at the end of most *Workbook* chapters. Every report is assigned at least once, with all answers being provided in the corresponding *Workbook* chapter answer key.

1. EMERGENCY DEPARTMENT REPORT

The patient is a 32-year-old G-5, P-4, female at 36 weeks and 4 days by last menstrual period, who comes in to the emergency room complaining of a 4-day history of urinary frequency and urgency with cloudy urine. She is also complaining of some low back pain × 5 days. She denies burning, itching, pain with urination. She denies fever and chills. She has also had some nausea and vomiting over the same period. She last vomited yesterday. She vomited twice, she states, and, this past Friday, 4 days ago, twice. She has not vomited today. She has had good fluid intake. She has had a slightly decreased appetite, she states. The patient states that she has had some UTIs this pregnancy × 2. Otherwise, she has had an uncomplicated pregnancy.

The patient denies a history of hypertension, diabetes, and pre-eclampsia. She states she has had some irregular contractions, no real contractions today. She denies vaginal bleeding. She denies gush of fluid. She denies abdominal pain. She has had good fetal movement. She has not had headaches, visual changes, or abdominal pain.

PHYSICAL EXAMINATION: Blood pressure 119/66, temperature 36.5, pulse 86, respiratory rate 18. HEENT: Within normal limits. CHEST: Clear to auscultation bilaterally. HEART: Regular rate and rhythm without murmur, rub, or gallop. ABDOMEN: Gravida, nontender. Vertex. EXTREMITIES: The patient has 1+ pitting edema bilaterally to the knee. On cervical examination, the patient was 1-2 cm, long, −1 station. Fetal heart tones are 130's with accels. *(average fetal heart rate is 120-160, so this is not an abnormal rate)* No obvious contractions on the monitor. No flank tenderness to palpation.

Copyright © 2016 by Elsevier Inc.

LABORATORY DATA: Urinalysis is done and revealed yellow, turbid urine, specific gravity of 1.022, 100 protein, positive nitrite, moderate hemoglobin, large amount of leukocytes, 5-10 red cells, 3+ bacteria, too numerous to count white cells.

ASSESSMENT: This is a 32-year-old, G-5, P-4 at 36 and 4/5 weeks, with a urinary tract infection. The patient was given a prescription for Macrobid 100 mg p.o. b.i.d. × 7 days. She is instructed to follow up with her OB doctor in 2 days for recheck of her urine and her symptomatology. She was given labor precautions. She was advised that, if she develops fevers, back pain, worsening symptomatology, she should come in immediately for evaluation.

2. DISCHARGE SUMMARY

DIAGNOSES include:

1. Chronic pelvic pain secondary to pelvic metastatic clear cell carcinoma of unknown primary location.
2. Vena cava syndrome post placement of Hickman catheter.
3. Anemia due to chronic disease.
4. Hypertension.

HOSPITAL COURSE: The patient is a 78-year-old female whom we have been following in our clinic for hypertension and also chronic pudendal nerve pain. She had been recently diagnosed with pelvic metastatic clear cell carcinoma, which her primary location is unknown at this time. She will be discussing this further after the pathology reports are read. During her hospital stay a Hickman catheter was placed in order to have IV access for pain medication or future cancer therapy. She was also admitted for chronic pain. She did develop swelling of her arms and neck. She was brought to interventional radiology and she did have venography and the Hickman catheter was removed. Her swelling to her arms and neck have decreased greatly. She denies any shortness of breath. No choking sensation as previously noted. Her pain has been managed well with fentanyl patch at 175 mcg. She has also been on IV heparin therapy for anticoagulation following the vena cava syndrome. Today, the patient has been having complaints of nausea. She did get some dexamethasone IV for her nausea, which did improve later this morning. Her blood pressure has been under good control. Her labs today include a WBC of 5.18, hemoglobin 7.8, hematocrit 23.7, protime 14.4, INR 1.5, PTT 39.6, BUN 6, sodium 139, potassium 4.2, CO_2 27.2.

DISCHARGE PLANS:

1. IV heparin is discontinued. She will be switched over to Lovenox 1 mg/kg subcutaneously daily. The patient will have Home Health to help her set up these injections.
2. She will continue with the fentanyl patch 175 mcg for the pain.
3. She will receive 40,000 units subcutaneously of Procrit at the Cancer Center one time per week. We will follow up in 3 days with a CBC and a basic metabolic panel.
4. Follow-up appointment at the Hypertension Center on November 2 at 10:30 in the morning. Will also check CBC and a basic metabolic panel, PTT, PT, and INR before that appointment.
5. Hold potassium supplements for now.
6. She may use Phenergan p.o. 12.5 mg 1-2 tablets p.o. p.r.n. every 6 hours for nausea.

Copyright © 2016 by Elsevier Inc.

7. She does have a follow-up appointment set up with Dr. Smith on Friday, 10/29/XX, to discuss her pathology results and decide what further treatment is to be done. He will also be discussing plans with Dr. Sticca.

The above plan was discussed with the patient and her husband. They seem to be in agreement. They were encouraged to call our office with any questions or concerns.

DISCHARGE MEDICATIONS:

1. Will continue home medications.
2. Phenergan 12.5 1-2 tabs p.o. p.r.n. every 6 hours for nausea.
3. Lovenox 1 mg/kg subcutaneously every 24 hours. *(treatment for thrombosis—blood clots)*
4. Fentanyl patch 175 mcg to be changed every 3 days. *(analgesic)*
5. Epogen 40,000 units subcutaneously weekly at the Cancer Center. *(treatment for anemia)*

Total time spent with the patient today is 60 minutes.

3. CLINIC CHART NOTE

HISTORY: This 16-year-old female is seen today after falling off a curb and twisting her right ankle. She is normally a patient of Dr. Anderson, who is out of town this week. *(Both physicians are of the same specialty and in the same clinic.)* She states that she has pain surrounding the entire foot and ankle. Seems unable or unwilling to bear weight. *(Problem focused history)*

PHYSICAL EXAMINATION: Ankle and foot examined. Foot is warm to touch. Some swelling and bruising noted around the lateral aspect of the ankle. X-ray is negative for fracture. (Problem focused examination)

IMPRESSION: Sprained right ankle. (MDM complexity straightforward)

PLAN: Elevation; ice to affected area. Weight bearing only as tolerated. Return for follow-up p.r.n.

4. ADMIT INPATIENT

This is a 19-year-old with a living-related donor kidney transplant as of last month and admitted to hospital for possible sepsis.

HISTORY: This patient has type 1 diabetes and had been on dialysis for a number of years before transplantation. She received her mother's kidney on the 14th of last month from the Medical Center Transplant Program in Dallas. She was there this Tuesday for a transplant visit and apparently did not feel well, but they were not certain whether this was a problem or not; but they did go ahead and do blood cultures and called the public health nurse, who was visiting the patient today, and said that one of the cultures was positive for group B strep. The home health nurse called me and stated that the patient has really gone downhill the past few days and was quite fatigued with generalized malaise. Denied cough, fever, or shaking chills but looked poor overall, and the nurse was quite concerned. We recommended she be brought here for evaluation and treatment as an emergency. After arrival here, she was in no acute distress. Initially, she had bibasilar crackles on deep breathing; however, most of these cleared. I cannot hear any significant pulmonary abnormality on auscultation or percussion. Her heart is normal regular rhythm. No significant murmurs, rubs, S3, or S4. Her

Copyright © 2016 by Elsevier Inc.

abdomen is negative. Her left lower-quadrant kidney is nontender. She has no edema and no lateralizing neural sounds. She is a little lethargic. She does not feel warm. Apparently she is afebrile. Her blood pressure is normal, and she is not tachycardic, but she simply does not look well. Past history, social history, and system review are per our recent old chart and noncontributory at present.

MEDICATIONS: See med sheet.

CLINICAL IMPRESSION: One positive group B strep blood culture, significance, and/or etiology to be determined. My impression at this time is probably a significant finding, and I suspect that this will become a progressive syndrome if not treated.

ADDITIONAL DIAGNOSES:

1. Living-related donor kidney transplant
2. Diabetes mellitus type 1
3. Hypertension

PLAN: Repeat culture. Culture urine. Do chest x-ray stat and repeat lab. Will empirically treat pending results at this time.

5. NEPHROLOGY HOSPITAL PROGRESS NOTE

This patient continues to be stable with no new problems. Her cultures remain negative, and she remains afebrile. Her clearance is pending, but she certainly has settled down nicely. The main problem we are having is with her diabetic management. It simply is not working with the former twice a day of 70/30 insulin plus a nighttime Lantus. I think we should go one way or the other, and we will go to Humalog before each meal, starting with an estimated dose of 15 per meal and 40 of Lantus in the evening, and we will titrate from there. We will get Accu-Cheks before each meal to reflect the previous meal's dose of Humalog and adjust it accordingly. Other than that, tomorrow we will review her case with infectious disease with regard to the duration of her antibiotic therapy. Thus far, our cultures have remained negative; however, the positive group B strep is not the type of typical contaminant you get in a blood culture, and we must take it at face value.

Time spent re-evaluating the patient, reviewing the chart, and rearranging diabetic management was 25 minutes; more than half of the time was coordination.

6. OPERATIVE REPORT

PREOPERATIVE DIAGNOSIS: Scar right parietal region.

POSTOPERATIVE DIAGNOSIS: Same.

SURGICAL FINDINGS: 3 × 1 cm elevated scar right parietal region of scalp.

SURGICAL PROCEDURE: Excision scar of scalp.

SURGEON: Dr. Harold Wallingford

ANESTHESIA: General endotracheal anesthesia, plus 2 cc of 1% Xylocaine and 1:100,000 epinephrine.

Copyright © 2016 by Elsevier Inc.

PROCEDURE: The scalp was prepped with Betadine scrub and solution, draped in the routine sterile fashion. The lesion was anesthetized with 2 cc of 1% Xylocaine with 1:100,000 epinephrine, mostly for the epinephrine effect. After a wait of 4 minutes the lesion was excised, bleeding was electrocoagulated, the wound was closed with vertical mattress sutures of 3-0 Prolene. Surgicel and antibiotic ointment were applied. The patient tolerated the procedure well and left the operating room in good condition.

PATHOLOGY REPORT LATER INDICATED: Benign tissue.

7. OPERATIVE REPORT

PREOPERATIVE DIAGNOSIS: Lipoma left posterior axillary fold.

POSTOPERATIVE DIAGNOSIS: Same.

SURGICAL FINDINGS: 6 cm diameter lipoma attached to latissimus dorsi muscle.

PROCEDURE PERFORMED: Excision of lipoma left posterior axillary fold.

ANESTHESIA: General endotracheal anesthesia with 5 cc 1% Xylocaine with 1:100,000 epinephrine injected along the incision line.

COMPLICATIONS: None.

SPONGE AND NEEDLE COUNT: Correct.

DRAINS: One #10 Jackson Pratt.

DESCRIPTION OF PROCEDURE: The patient's posterior arm was prepped with Betadine scrub and solution and draped in the routine sterile fashion. About 5 cc of 1% Xylocaine with 1:100,000 epinephrine were injected along the incision line. Dissection was carried down to the site of the lipomatous mass, which was dissected free of the skin and dissected free of the muscle using sharp dissection with very little bleeding. Bleeding was electrocoagulated. Because of the size of the pocket, we inserted a drain and brought it out through a separate stab wound incision using a #10 Jackson Pratt drain. The wound was then closed, effectively closing the dead space with interrupted 2-0 Monocryl, subcuticular 3-0 Monocryl, and a few twists of 4-0 Prolene. Dressing consisted of Kerlix fluffs, Elastoplast, a clavicle strap, and a sling. The patient tolerated the procedure well and left the area in good condition.

PATHOLOGY REPORT LATER INDICATED: See Report 60.

8. OPERATIVE REPORT

PREOPERATIVE DIAGNOSIS: Pyogenic granuloma, sinus tract, buttock.

POSTOPERATIVE DIAGNOSIS: Multiple sinus tracts, one extending inferiorly about 7 × 3 cm in diameter, one extending to the right approximately 4 × 3 cm, and one 4 × 3 cm extending to the left of 4 × 3 cm.

SURGICAL FINDINGS: As above, plus (benign) granulation tissue present in a capsule of multiple sinus tracts. Sinus tracts measured a total of about 15 × 8 cm in their total dimensions.

Copyright © 2016 by Elsevier Inc.

SURGICAL PROCEDURE: Partial unroofing of sinus tracts. *(This is a full-thickness debridement.)*

ANESTHESIA: General endotracheal.

DESCRIPTION OF PROCEDURE: The patient was intubated and turned in the prone position. A probe was inserted in the sinus cavity, and dissection was carried down to this. I encountered a piece of chronically infected granulation tissue coming out of a hole, in which I stuck the probe, but this continued for a distance longer than the probe and accordingly, I put my finger in this and this extended down the length of my index finger *(i.e., about 7-8 cm by about 3 cm in width)*. I left this intact, because this would necessitate extensive dissection of 15 sq. cm. of subcutaneous tissue and we have no blood on this patient at this time. We then unroofed two other sinus cavities, and packed this opened with 2-inch vaginal packing and applied a dressing and Kerlix plus an Elastoplast. Estimated blood loss: 25 cc. The patient seemed to tolerate the procedure well and left the operating room in good condition.

   Coder's Query: It is unclear from the documentation exactly what the procedure was that the physician performed. The coder queried the physician and asked for additional information to ensure correct coding. The physician explained that the patient has a recurrent history of pyogenic granuloma of the buttock with sinus tracts that have, as in this instance, required a subcutaneous tissue debridement.

9. OPERATIVE REPORT

PREOPERATIVE DIAGNOSIS: Mass, right breast.

POSTOPERATIVE DIAGNOSIS: Mass, right breast.

OPERATIVE PROCEDURE: Right breast mass excision.

PROCEDURE: With the female patient under general anesthesia, the breast and chest were prepped and draped in a sterile manner. An elliptical incision was made in the central portion of the breast about the palpated mass, including the area of the nipple. This was excised all the way down to the fascia of the breast and then submitted for frozen section. Frozen section revealed a carcinoma of the breast with what appeared to be a good margin all the way around it. We then maintained hemostasis with electrocautery and proceeded to close the breast tissue using 2-0 and 3-0 chromic. The skin was closed using 4-0 Vicryl in a subcuticular manner. Steri-Strips were applied. The patient tolerated the procedure well and was discharged from the operating room in stable condition.

PATHOLOGY REPORT LATER INDICATED: Primary, malignant neoplasm.

10. OPERATIVE REPORT

PREOPERATIVE DIAGNOSIS: Neck injury, closed posterior cord syndrome caused by a fracture due to a motor vehicle accident.

POSTOPERATIVE DIAGNOSIS: Same as preoperative.

PROCEDURE PERFORMED: Placement of halo crown and vest.

ANESTHESIA: Local.

Copyright © 2016 by Elsevier Inc.

SURGICAL INDICATIONS: This 56-year-old patient was in a motor vehicle accident, hitting a tree. He was the driver and appears to have sustained a cervical spinal cord fracture at C1–4. He could not be placed in a neck collar because he has a short, thick neck and also because he had a tracheostomy tube. The patient would not be stabilized with traction as he has a distraction injury. It was indicated to place him in a halo vest and crown to immobilize his neck.

PROCEDURE: The hair was shaved behind both ears. There was a sterile prep done along the forehead region and the region behind both ears. The halo crown was then positioned and stabilized with the three positioners anteriorly and two laterally. I then injected Xylocaine behind both ears and along the supraorbital ridge laterally. I then placed the four pins and torqued them to 8 pounds per sq inch. The hexagonal lock nuts were then tightened. The patient tolerated this well without any apparent complications. The halo vest was then connected to the crown. The crown was placed. A large vest was used but this was still too small for the patient, and on the right side the vest had to be tied with string until some permanent straps could be fashioned by orthotics. During the placement of the vest, I maintained the neck in neutral position and at no time was there any rotation or flexion or extension of the neck.

11. OPERATIVE REPORT

PREOPERATIVE DIAGNOSIS: Bulky free flap, right heel.

POSTOPERATIVE DIAGNOSIS: Same.

SURGICAL FINDINGS: 10.5 × 8.5 cm area of redundant fat of flap of right heel.

PROCEDURE PERFORMED: Defatting of flap of right heel with excision of redundant skin (benign).

ANESTHESIA: General endotracheal anesthesia.

POSITION: Prone.

ESTIMATED BLOOD LOSS: Negligible.

DESCRIPTION OF PROCEDURE: The patient was intubated and turned into prone position. The right foot and lower leg were prepped with Betadine scrub and solution and was draped in the routine sterile fashion. The medial aspect of the flap was elevated excising the old scar in the process, and the flap was elevated to about 60% of its extent to include all of the redundant fat that was within the flap. We removed about 1.5 cm thickness of flap from the bottom of the flap and left a layer of padding of about a cm on the bed. Hemostasis was secured, and then we closed the wound with a combination of plain 3-0 Prolene and horizontal mattress sutures and some horizontal half mattress sutures of 3-0 Prolene. We dressed the wound temporarily with Kerlix and Kling. Dr. Miller will then proceed with his portion of the procedure.

12. OPERATIVE REPORT

PREOPERATIVE DIAGNOSIS: Ischial pressure ulcer with massive ischioperineal and buttock sinus.

Copyright © 2016 by Elsevier Inc.

POSTOPERATIVE DIAGNOSIS: Same.

FINDINGS: There was a 2 cm open surgical ulcer extending down and connecting with an 8 × 30 cm diameter granulation-lined sinus cavity.

SURGICAL PROCEDURE: Excision of left ischial ulcer with total excision of 8 × 30 cm sinus of the buttock, perineal, and ischial areas.

ANESTHESIA: General endotracheal.

ESTIMATED BLOOD LOSS: 400 ml.

FLUIDS: 2 liters Ringer's lactate.

DRAINS: None.

COMPLICATION: None.

SPONGE AND NEEDLE COUNTS: Correct.

DESCRIPTION: The patient was intubated and turned in the right lateral decubitus position. I injected about 10 ml of 1% Xylocaine with 1 : 100,000 epinephrine around the surface ulcer, and made incisions down to the granulation tissue, keeping this intact. I opened the skin over the extent of the sinus tracts proximally and distally, trying to keep this in line with a potential Y-V advancement flap, and with some difficulty and remarkable bleeding around what appeared to be the sacrum, I was able to remove virtually intact the entire ulcer, covered with chronically infected granulation tissue. This granulation tissue was poor quality and had an unhealthy appearance. A piece of this was dropped in a culture tube as was a piece of what appeared to be the sacrum, which was quite sclerotic and consistent with an osteomyelitis of the sacrum. Following this extensive removal of the ulcer, I cauterized all of the bleeding and did a stick-tie on one of the bleeders with 2-0 Vicryl. I then sprayed the base with topical thrombin, packed the wound open with 2-inch vaginal packing soaked in 5/10th percent metronidazole, and then put several #2 Prolene sutures to keep the packing in place and to help seal off the wound from the fecal contamination. I put a Vi-Drape over this and then dressed it with Kerlix fluffs, ABD pads, and Elastoplast. The patient tolerated the procedure well and left the area in good condition.

PATHOLOGY REPORT LATER INDICATED: See Report 62.

13. OPERATIVE REPORT

PROCEDURE: Steroid injection.

INDICATIONS: Left shoulder bursitis, rotator cuff syndrome.

PROCEDURE: This procedure was done in the procedure area in the outpatient department of the hospital. After obtaining consent, area of the left shoulder was prepped in the usual fashion with Betadine. 6 cc of 1% lidocaine with 1 cc of Kenalog was injected in the left subacromial bursa without difficulty. The patient tolerated the procedure well without immediate complications. There was moderate relief of pain afterward. The patient was advised to call me if she gets any signs of infection, such as fever, chills, erythema, or swelling. She will call me in 3 days and tell me how she is doing.

Copyright © 2016 by Elsevier Inc.

14. OPERATIVE REPORT

PREOPERATIVE DIAGNOSIS: Deltoid muscle pain and swelling, myositis.

POSTOPERATIVE DIAGNOSIS: Same.

PRELIMINARY NOTE: This patient was brought down to the operating room on the ventilator, and we used the operating room because of this.

OPERATIVE NOTE: With the patient in the supine position we prepped and draped the left deltoid region. After infiltration with 0.5% Marcaine with epinephrine, a vertical incision was made over the palpated muscular belly. Sharp dissection was carried down to the muscle belly and then we freed up a segment of muscle. We did infiltrate the ends of the muscle away from where we were taking our biopsy with the Marcaine. A segment of muscle was then isolated between clamps and then we excised the segment of muscle and submitted it immediately to the histology department for proper processing. The ends of the muscle were ligated using 2-0 chromic and then the muscular fascia was brought together using 2-0 chromic. Subcutaneous tissue was closed using 2-0 chromic and then the skin was closed using 4-0 nylon in running mattress fashion. A sterile dressing was applied. The patient tolerated the procedure well and was discharged from the operating room in stable condition. At the end of the procedure all sponges and instruments were accounted for.

PATHOLOGY REPORT LATER INDICATED: See Report 59.

15. OPERATIVE REPORT

PREOPERATIVE DIAGNOSIS: Left distal radius fracture.

POSTOPERATIVE DIAGNOSIS: Same.

PROCEDURE PERFORMED: Closed reduction and pinning of closed left distal radius fracture.

COMPLICATIONS: None.

INDICATIONS: This is a 31-year-old female who fell yesterday down a flight of stairs, fracturing her left wrist. She has been stabilized in the intensive care unit throughout the day today. Her injuries include a comminuted intra-articular left distal radius fracture, displaced.
The patient's x-rays are consistent with a displaced comminuted intra-articular distal radius fracture. This is an unstable fracture and requires reduction and probable pinning versus open reduction and internal fixation.

Prior to the procedure, I spoke with the patient regarding her left wrist. We discussed management options in detail, and I recommended proceeding with a closed reduction versus pinning versus ORIF of her left distal radius. The procedure, alternatives, risks, benefits, and expected rehab course were discussed in detail. She understood the implications of surgery and wished to proceed.

PROCEDURE: The patient was brought to the operating room and placed supine on the operating room table. She underwent general anesthesia. The left wrist was initially examined under fluoroscopic guidance. There was comminution and intra-articular involvement. There was dorsal tilt of 30

Copyright © 2016 by Elsevier Inc.

degrees, shortening, and angulation. We performed a closed reduction with longitudinal traction, manipulation at the fracture, and volar flexion. We obtained a near anatomic reduction with maintenance of radial length and inclination. Additionally, there was neutral tilt. However, with release of traction, there was some instability to the fracture with some residual collapse. Subsequently, the left upper extremity was prepped and draped in standard surgical fashion. Under fluoroscopic guidance, a closed reduction was again obtained. Two separate 0.062 K-wires were placed through the radial styloid, across the main fracture, and into the more proximal shaft. Both of these screws had good fixation in the bone.

Final fluoroscopic views were obtained confirming a near anatomic reduction. The pins were then cut off 1 cm above skin level. The pin sites were dressed with Xeroform gauze and adequately padded. The left upper extremity was then placed into a well-padded and molded long arm cast with the wrist in neutral, forearm neutral, and elbow 90 degrees.

The patient was awakened from anesthesia and tolerated the procedure well. She was transferred back to the recovery room in stable condition. There were no intraoperative complications for the wrist portion of the procedure.

16. OPERATIVE REPORT

PREOPERATIVE DIAGNOSIS: Degenerative joint disease, medial compartment plus old meniscal tear.

POSTOPERATIVE DIAGNOSIS: Posterior horn tear, old, medial meniscus; diffuse grade 3-4 chondromalacia, medial femoral condyle 0-90 degrees; and grade 4 chondromalacia, superior half of the patella.

PROCEDURE PERFORMED: Arthroscopy and partial arthroscopic meniscectomy, right knee.

OPERATIVE PROCEDURE: After suitable general anesthesia had been achieved, the patient's right knee was prepped and draped in the usual manner. Before prepping, a thigh tourniquet was applied; after draping, it was inflated to 300 mm Hg. No inflow cannula was used. Arthroscope was inserted through an anteromedial portal. The lateral compartment was examined. Everything looked good. Examination of the notch revealed some inflated synovial tissue, which was cauterized with a radiofrequency probe. Examination of the medial compartment revealed a horizontal cleavage tear and flap tear of the posterior horn of the medial meniscus. Using a combination of punch and shaver, the unstable meniscus was excised and contoured. The tibial surfaces revealed a small area of water by the anterior horn of the meniscus. Femoral surfaces showed diffuse wear of grade 3 with occasional areas of grade 4 chondromalacia from 0 to 90 degrees. Examination of the patellofemoral joint revealed very good looking articular surfaces on the inferior half of the patella in the trochlea. However, there was essentially bare bone on the superior half of the articular surface.

The knee joint was then thoroughly irrigated, and the arthroscope removed. Stab wounds were closed with 3-0 nylon. A dressing was then applied. Tourniquet was released, after which good circulation was noted to return to the foot. The patient tolerated the procedure well and returned to the recovery room in stable condition.

PATHOLOGY REPORT LATER INDICATED: Benign meniscus tissue and bone chips.

Copyright © 2016 by Elsevier Inc.

17. OPERATIVE REPORT

PREOPERATIVE DIAGNOSIS: Subtrochanteric fracture, closed, right hip.

POSTOPERATIVE DIAGNOSIS: Subtrochanteric fracture, right hip.

PROCEDURE PERFORMED: Open reduction internal fixation of subtrochanteric fracture, right hip.

ANESTHESIA: Spinal.

FINDINGS: The patient had a displaced comminuted subtrochanteric fracture of her right hip. We were able to align this fairly well and hold this in place with a dynamic hip screw device.

PROCEDURE: While under spinal anesthetic, the patient was placed in the supine position on the fracture table, where gentle traction was applied to the right leg and the left leg was abducted. We visualized the fracture using the C-arm image intensifier. We were satisfied with the position and then prepped the patient's right hip with Betadine and draped it in a sterile fashion. She was given 1 g of Kefzol intravenously preoperatively.

We then created a longitudinal incision over the lateral aspect of the right hip and carried the dissection down through the subcutaneous tissue. The fascia was incised longitudinally, and we reflected the vastus lateralis anteriorly, exposing the lateral aspect of the femoral shaft. We were able to palpate the fracture and found that it was significantly displaced. We attempted to reduce this. We then drilled a 9/64-inch hole in the lateral aspect of the femoral shaft through which we advanced a guide pin into the femoral head at an angle of 135 degrees to the femoral shaft. We then passed a reamer over this and reamed to a depth of 110 mm and inserted a 100-mg lag screw into the femoral head. We attempted to position this lag screw in the center of the femoral head as best as possible as seen in both the AP and lateral views.

We then attached a 135-degree four-hole side plate and secured this plate to the femoral shaft using four cortical screws. We then released the traction of the leg and inserted a compressing screw into the end of the lag screw. The resultant fixation appeared to be quite satisfactory. We again used the C-arm image intensifier to evaluate the fracture and found it to be very acceptable.

We then thoroughly irrigated the area with saline and placed a Hemovac drain deep to the fascia. We then closed the fascia using 0 Vicryl and the subcutaneous tissue with 2-0 Vicryl. The skin was closed using skin staples. A sterile Xeroform dressing was applied, and the patient was then taken from the operating room in good condition breathing spontaneously. The final sponge and needle counts were correct. She will be continued on IV Kefzol for at least 24 hours.

18. OPERATIVE REPORT

PREOPERATIVE DIAGNOSIS: Comminuted fracture, right olecranon process of the ulna.

POSTOPERATIVE DIAGNOSIS: Comminuted fracture, right olecranon process of the ulna.

PROCEDURE PERFORMED: Open reduction internal fixation, right olecranon fracture.

Copyright © 2016 by Elsevier Inc.

ANESTHESIA: General.

FINDINGS: The patient had a markedly comminuted displaced fracture of his right olecranon. He had involved a significant portion of the articular surface. We were able to reassemble the major fragments; however, we did have to debride some of the articular cartilage from the joint, which resulted in a defect in the articular cartilage of some significance.

PROCEDURE: While under a general anesthetic, the patient was placed in supine position on the operating room table, where his right arm was prepped with Betadine and draped in a sterile fashion. We used an Esmarch bandage to exsanguinate the arm, and a tourniquet on the limb was inflated to 250 mm Hg. The total tourniquet time ended up being 43 minutes.

We created a longitudinal incision over the posterior aspect of the elbow, skirting to the radial side of the olecranon. We carried the dissection down through the subcutaneous tissue and easily identified the fracture site as the periosteum was torn over this area. We used suction to irrigate the hematoma. Several pieces of articular cartilage lay in the joint, which we debrided, and there was some other cancellous bone, which we debrided as well because it was laying loose in the joint. We then thoroughly irrigated the area with saline to look for any remaining loose fragments. We held this in place with a towel clip as we drilled a transverse hole through the ulna, perhaps 2.5 cm distal to the fracture site. We passed an 18-gauge wire through this transverse tunnel through the ulna, and then we passed two smooth Steinmann pins across the fracture site. We started the Steinmann pins from the proximal fragment and drilled across the fracture site into the distal ulnar shaft. After we had completed the second Steinmann pin across the fracture site, we passed the 18-gauge wire in a figure-of-eight fashion across the fracture site and around the Steinmann pins. We then tightened this with a Harris wire tightener. The combination of the Steinmann pins and the figure-of-eight wire seemed to secure the fracture quite nicely. There was no movement of the fracture site with placing the elbow through a range of motion. We left the Steinmann pins long until we had obtained an intraoperative x-ray confirming an acceptable alignment of the fragment. The x-rays did confirm a significant loss of the articular cartilage; however, it was elected to accept this because the fragments appeared to be relatively stable clinically.

We then bent the Steinmann pins at 90 degrees and cut them off and then taped the Steinmann pins so that they were buried into the triceps muscle. We placed the elbow through a range of motion and found that no crepitus was noted. The fracture appeared to be in good condition, and we therefore irrigated the area with saline and closed the subcutaneous tissue using 2-0 Vicryl and the skin with 3-0 nylon. A Xeroform dressing was applied, and a long-arm splint was applied with the elbow flexed about 60 degrees. He was taken from the operating room in good condition and breathing spontaneously. Tourniquet released after 43 minutes of tourniquet time, and we released this just after the x-rays. He was given IV Kefzol preoperatively and will be continued on IV Kefzol for 24 hours postoperatively as well. The final sponge and needle counts were correct.

19. OPERATIVE REPORT

PREOPERATIVE DIAGNOSIS: Left lung abscess.

POSTOPERATIVE DIAGNOSIS: Same.

Copyright © 2016 by Elsevier Inc.

PROCEDURE PERFORMED: Left upper lobectomy with decortication and drainage.

INDICATIONS: This 52-year-old female with radiographic evidence of a left upper lobe abscess was admitted the evening before surgery with tension pneumothorax treated with double-lumen intubation and a chest tube. She was subsequently dialyzed to improve hemodynamics and oxygenation and was felt to be as optimal as possible for her left thoracotomy.

FINDINGS AT SURGERY revealed a large abscess in the left upper lobe accounting for approximately 70% of the left upper lobe parenchyma. Fibrinopurulent exudate was noted on the left lower lobe and throughout the parietal pleural surfaces. This was removed piecemeal with gradual improvement in the left lower lobe pulmonary expansion.

PROCEDURE: The patient was brought to the operating room and placed in the supine position, and under general intubation with a double-lumen tube that had been placed the night before, the patient was rolled into the right lateral decubitus position with her left side up. A posterolateral thoracotomy was performed. Adhesions were taken down sharply and bluntly and with cautery. Following this, a standard artery first left upper lobectomy was carried out utilizing 0 silk and hemoclips. The left upper pulmonary vein was secured with a single application of the TA-30 vascular stapling machine. The posterior fissure was created with multiple applications of the TIA automatic stapling machine and the bronchus secured with a single application of the TA-30 bronchus stapling machine. Following this, the wound was drained with three 24-French atrium chest tubes and hemostasis obtained with spray Tisseel, Surgicel gauze. The bronchus was sealed with Bio-glue and the wound closed in layers and a sterile compression dressing applied, and the patient returned to the surgical intensive care unit after changing the double-lumen tube to a single-lumen tube. The patient received 3 units of packed cells intraoperatively to maintain hemostasis. Sponge count and needle count correct × 2.

PATHOLOGY REPORT LATER INDICATED: See Report 65.

20. OPERATIVE REPORT

Endocervical and Endometrial Biopsy

The patient is a 60-year-old married white female, whose last menstrual period was at age 55. No postmenopausal bleeding. Pap is current. Mammogram is not given.

CHIEF COMPLAINT: Metastatic clear cell carcinoma.

The patient is status post CT-guided transgluteal biopsy of a presacral mass, which returns as metastatic clear cell carcinoma. Biopsy was performed September 17, 20XX. The patient's CT of the abdomen shows the uterus to be slightly enlarged for patient's age but does not mention ascites or ovarian masses.

MEDICATIONS:

1. Citracal.
2. Lanoxin 0.25 mg.
3. Metoprolol 50 mg b.i.d.
4. Multivitamin.

Copyright © 2016 by Elsevier Inc.

5. Ocuvite.
6. Xanax.

MEDICAL PROBLEMS:

1. Chronic pelvic pain syndrome.
2. Sacroiliac lipoma.
3. Pudendal neuralgia.
4. Hiatal hernia.

FAMILY HISTORY: Negative.

REVIEW OF SYSTEMS: Positive for glasses, high blood pressure, anxiety, depression.

PROCEDURE: Endocervical and endometrial biopsy.

The patient received antibiotic prophylaxis and then the procedure was performed by visualizing the cervix. The cervix was prepped with Betadine, and cytobrush was then used to obtain cervical curetting. The endocervical os was unable to be demonstrated by the Pipelle curette or the uterine sound. The cytobrush was then used to locate the central endometrial canal, and the Pipelle curette was then used to obtain endometrial curetting. Bimanual examination shows the uterus to measure 4 to 6 weeks, anteverted, smooth, mobile. Adnexa negative. Rectal declined. BUS within normal limits.

IMPRESSION: Clear cell carcinoma of unknown origin.

PLAN: Refer the patient to the University of Minnesota for diagnostic workup and treatment. The patient and University of Minnesota will be advised of the results of the biopsies when they become available.

PATHOLOGY REPORT LATER INDICATED: See Report 54.

21. OPERATIVE REPORT

PREOPERATIVE DIAGNOSIS: Atelectasis of the right lower lobe, suspecting either a mucous plug or obstructing cancer.

POSTOPERATIVE DIAGNOSIS: Mildly inflamed airways with some thick secretions. No definite mucous plug was seen, and certainly no cancer was noted.

PROCEDURE PERFORMED: Bronchoalveolar lavage, bronchial brushings, and bronchial washings.

For a detail of drugs used and amounts of drugs used, please refer to the bronchoscopy report sheet.

The patient was in the ICU on the ventilator, intubated, and so we simply used ICU sedation. We put the bronchoscope down the endotracheal tube. We could see the trachea, which appeared okay. The carina appeared normal. In the right and left lungs, all segments were patent and entered, and in the right lower lobe and middle lower lobe, there were increased, thick, tenacious secretions. No definite mucous plug. It did take a little suctioning to dislodge all of the mucus; however, it was not as bad as I thought it would be looking at the x-ray. The area was brushed, washed, and then, to be more specific, because of evidence on chest x-ray of something going on in the periphery, a bronchoalveolar lavage of the right lower lobe is performed. The patient tolerated the procedure well. Specimens were performed. Specimens were sent for appropriate cytological, pathological, and bacteriological studies, and we hope to be able to follow up on that tomorrow.

PATHOLOGY REPORT LATER INDICATED: See Report 66.

Copyright © 2016 by Elsevier Inc.

22. OPERATIVE REPORT

PREOPERATIVE DIAGNOSIS: Chronic adenotonsillitis and chronic tonsillitis.

POSTOPERATIVE DIAGNOSIS: Chronic adenotonsillitis and chronic tonsillitis.

PROCEDURE PERFORMED: Tonsillectomy and adenoidectomy.

OPERATIVE NOTE: The patient is a 15-year-old woman who was seen in the office and diagnosed with the above condition. Decision was made in consultation with the patient to undergo the procedure.

She was admitted through the same-day department and taken to the operating room, where she was administered general anesthetic by intravenous injection. She was then intubated endotracheally. The Jennings gag was inserted into the mouth and expanded; this was secured to a Mayo stand. Two red rubber catheters were placed through the nose and brought out through the mouth; these were secured with snaps. This was done to elevate the palate. A laryngeal mirror was placed in the nasopharynx. The adenoid tissue was visualized. Using suction cautery, the adenoid tissue was removed in systemic fashion. Once this was completed, the red rubbers were released and brought out through the nose. The right tonsil was grasped with an Allis forceps and retracted medially using a harmonic scalpel, and the capsule was entered bilaterally. The tonsil was removed from its fossa in an inferior fashion, and one small area was cauterized. The left tonsil was then grasped with an Allis forceps and retracted medially. Again, the capsule was identified laterally, and the harmonic scalpel was used to remove the tonsil from its fossa in an inferior to superior fashion. Once this was completed, the bed was inspected, and two small areas were cauterized here. Three tonsillar sponges were soaked in 1% Marcaine with epinephrine; one was placed in the nasopharynx, and one in each tonsil bed. These were left in position for 5 minutes, and at the end of this interval they were removed. The beds were inspected. No further bleeding was noted. The gag was then removed from the mouth. The TMJ joint was checked. The patient was allowed to recover from a general anesthetic and taken to the post anesthesia care unit in stable condition. There were no complications during this procedure.

PATHOLOGY REPORT LATER INDICATED: Benign tonsil and adenoid tissue.

23. OPERATIVE REPORT

PREOPERATIVE DIAGNOSIS: Pleural fluid, unknown cause.

POSTOPERATIVE DIAGNOSIS: Loculated pleural effusion with removal of 40 cc of bloody pleural fluid.

PROCEDURE PERFORMED: Diagnostic thoracentesis.

On ultrasound, the areas were loculated by that method as well as by attempting to draw out fluid. I had to do four different sticks to get 40 cc of fluid and that was about the extent of each pocket. There were four different pockets I entered just in the one general area that was marked by ultrasound. This, of course, was done after marking it with ultrasound, rubbing the area with swabs to sterilize the area, and then using 20 cc of 1% lidocaine for local anesthesia. With a one-pass maneuver, we were able to get into some fluid. At first actually, we did not get any fluid. We moved over about 1 inch, and then we were able to get 10 cc of fluid before the

Copyright © 2016 by Elsevier Inc.

pocket petered out. The next one we got 5 cc, and I had to go to a different pocket to get that. Then in the fourth pocket we were able to get two syringe fulls with 10 cc to get at least 40 cc of fluid. As this was such a tenuous area, I did not put a chest tube in to drain it because I did not think we would get anything that would amount to anything with the small chest tube I had at my command. I think we might need thoracoscopy to break up adhesions and drain it right. Of course, the differential of bloody pleural fluid includes tuberculosis, trauma, cancer, and pulmonary embolus. A V/Q scan would probably be pointless in this particular effort. I think I would wait to see what the cultures are before I went down the pulmonary embolus tree. I will have to get a hold of Dr. Marrot about CT surgery.

PATHOLOGY REPORT LATER INDICATED: See Report 67.

24. OPERATIVE REPORT

PROCEDURE PERFORMED: Fiberoptic bronchoscopy, bronchial biopsy, bronchial washings, bronchial brushings.

PREPROCEDURE DIAGNOSIS: Abnormal chest x-ray.

POSTPROCEDURE DIAGNOSIS: Inflammation in all lobes, pneumonia. With pleural plaquing consistent with possible candidiasis.

The patient was already on a ventilator, so the bronchoscope tube was introduced through the endotracheal tube. We saw 2.5 cm above the carina of the trachea, which was red and swollen, as was the carina. The right lung—all entrances were patent, but they were all swollen and red, with increased secretions. The left lung was even more involved, with more swelling and more edema and had bloody secretions, especially at the left base. This area from the carina all the way down to the smaller airways on the left side had shown white plaquing consistent with possible candidiasis. These areas were brushed, washed, biopsied. A biopsy specimen was also sent for tissue culture, as well as two biopsy specimens sent for pathology. Sheath brushings were also performed. The patient tolerated the procedure well, was still in the ICU, monitored throughout the procedure.

25. CARDIAC CATHETERIZATION REPORT

PROCEDURES PERFORMED: Left-sided heart catheterization, selective coronary angiography, and left ventriculography.

INDICATION: Chest pain and abnormal Cardiolite stress test.

COMPLICATIONS: None.

RESULTS:

I. HEMODYNAMICS: The left ventricular pressure before the LV-gram was 117/1 with an LVEDP of 4. After the LV-gram, it was 111/4 with an LVEDP of 10. The aortic pressure on pullback was 111/17.

II. LEFT VENTRICULOGRAPHY: The left ventriculography showed that the left ventricle was of normal size. There were no significant segmental wall motion abnormalities. The overall left ventricular systolic function was normal with an ejection fraction of better than 60%.

Copyright © 2016 by Elsevier Inc.

III. SELECTIVE CORONARY ANGIOGRAPHY:

A. RIGHT CORONARY ARTERY: The right coronary artery is a medium to large size dominant artery that has about 80% to 90% proximal/mid eccentric stenosis. The rest of the artery has only mild surface irregularities. The PDA and the posterolateral branches are small in size and have only mild surface irregularities.

B. LEFT MAIN CORONARY ARTERY: The left main has mild distal narrowing.

C. LEFT CIRCUMFLEX ARTERY: The left circumflex artery was a medium size, nondominant artery. It gave rise to a very high first obtuse marginal/intermedius, which was a bifurcating medium size artery that has only mild surface irregularities. The second obtuse marginal was also a medium size artery that has about 20% to 25% proximal narrowing. After that second obtuse marginal, the circumflex artery was a small size artery that has about 20% to 30% narrowing, a small aneurysmal segment. After that, it continued as a small third obtuse marginal that has mild atherosclerotic disease.

D. LEFT ANTERIOR DESCENDING CORONARY ARTERY: The left anterior descending artery was a medium size artery that is mildly calcified. It gave rise to a very tiny first diagonal that has mild diffuse atherosclerotic disease. Right at the origin of the second diagonal, the LAD has about 30% narrowing. The rest of the artery was free of significant obstructive disease. The second diagonal was also a small caliber artery that has no significant obstructive disease.

CONCLUSION:

1. Normal overall left ventricular systolic function
2. Severe single vessel atherosclerotic heart disease

RECOMMENDATIONS: Angioplasty stent of the right coronary artery.

26. CORONARY ARTERY BYPASS SURGERY

PREOPERATIVE DIAGNOSIS: Atherosclerotic heart disease, coronary artery disease with depressed LV function.

POSTOPERATIVE DIAGNOSIS: Same.

PROCEDURE PERFORMED: Single vessel coronary artery bypass grafting, LIMA to LAD, off-pump.

ANESTHESIA: General endotracheal.

SPONGE COUNT, NEEDLE COUNT, INSTRUMENT COUNT: Correct.

ESTIMATED BLOOD LOSS: Approximately 666 cc and CellSaver given back is approximately 287 cc.

DRAINS: Four 19-French round Blake drains, one in the left chest, one in the right chest, one over the heart, and one over the pericardial wall, placed to Pleur-evac suction.

INDICATIONS: The patient is a 62-year-old man who has undergone approximately 12 heart catheterizations in the last several years. He has had recurrent in-stent stenosis of the proximal LAD lesion and also a branch of an OM with disease proximally. The patient is taken to the operating room because of recurrent angina, Class III anginal symptoms.

Copyright © 2016 by Elsevier Inc.

PROCEDURE: After informed consent was obtained, the patient was taken to the operating room. The patient was properly identified. A Swan-Ganz catheter was placed and a right arterial line was placed. A Foley catheter was inserted. The patient was prepped from his chin to both feet bilaterally. A midline sternotomy was performed. The sternum was divided with the sternal saw and the left internal mammary was harvested in a standard fashion.

Simultaneously, the right greater saphenous vein was harvested beginning in the thigh and extending down to the level of the knee. The vein was adequate for bypass grafting. It was excised. The wound was then closed in layers.

Once the LIMA was nearly completely dissected free, the patient was heparinized. The LIMA was divided distally and noted to have excellent flow. It was tied distally. LIMA bed was examined for bleeding. There appeared to be no bleeding present from the LIMA bed. Attention was then turned to the pericardium. The pericardium was opened. Pericardial stay sutures were placed. The left side of the pericardium was fashioned so that the LIMA could sit nicely to the LAD under the lung. Deep pericardial stitch was placed allowing the heart to be elevated and brought medially. A stay suture was placed around the proximal LAD and around the distal LAD. The octopus stabilizing device was used to stabilize the LAD at its mid portion. The proximal stay suture was placed down on the LAD. The LAD was opened and the LIMA had been fashioned for the anastomosis, and the LIMA to LAD anastomosis was carried out using a 7-0 Prolene in a continuous running fashion using a single knot technique. LIMA pedicle was then sutured down. There appeared to be no leak present from the LIMA anastomosis. The starfish stabilizing device was placed on the apex of the heart. The heart was elevated. The lateral wall of the heart was examined extensively for the OM branch that had some proximal disease in it. This artery was not able to be identified. The heart was covered heavily in fat making it somewhat more difficult, but a thorough examination was carried out. At this point I actually broke scrub, went to the catheterization laboratory, re-examined the heart catheterization, and then went back to the OR again looking for that vessel. It almost could have been acting like a high diagonal vessel as it was a high OM, but again in this territory in this distribution I could not identify that vessel, so only a single vessel LIMA to LAD anastomosis was created and the patient ended up with a single bypass. I think he should do well with just a single bypass.

The surgical sites were all examined for bleeding, and there appeared to be no bleeding present. The patient was reversed with 50 mg of Protamine and four Blake drains were placed, one in the left chest, one in the right chest, one over the heart, and one in the pericardial wall. The patient tolerated the procedure well. The preoperative and postoperative transesophageal echocardiogram looked fine. Sternal wires were placed and then the wound was closed in layers. Initial cardiac index here revealed a cardiac index of approximately 2.4 on low dose nitro drip.

27. OPERATIVE REPORT

PREOPERATIVE DIAGNOSIS: Symptomatic right internal carotid artery stenosis.

POSTOPERATIVE DIAGNOSIS: Symptomatic right internal carotid artery stenosis.

Copyright © 2016 by Elsevier Inc.

OPERATIVE PROCEDURE:

1. Right carotid thromboendarterectomy with patch placement.
2. Intraoperative electroencephalogram monitoring.

INDICATION: This 30-year-old woman has a tight right internal carotid artery stenosis. She has had an episode of amaurosis fugax. She has some other medical problems that also complicate her overall situation, but she has a significantly tight stenosis that is symptomatic, and I would recommend an endarterectomy for this. The procedure, along with the risks, has been previously discussed with the patient. Please see the clinic notes. We will be doing this with the patient awake. We also will be doing EEG monitoring though because of the patient's overall condition, and if she does not end up needing to be intubated during the middle of the case, we will still be able to monitor her brain activity.

PROCEDURE: This was done with the patient under cervical block. Local anesthesia was also infiltrated (0.5% Marcaine with epinephrine). Dissection was carried down through a cervical oblique incision along the anterior border of the sternocleidomastoid muscle. Dissection was carried down to the carotid artery. The common carotid as well as the internal and external carotid arteries and superior thyroid arteries were all dissected free sharply and circumferentially controlled with vessel loops. The common carotid was controlled with umbilical tape and Rumel tourniquet. The patient was systemically heparinized. ACTs were obtained and followed. The ICA was occluded, then the common and then the external carotid. Arteriotomy was made. The plaque was hemorrhagic and ulcerated. It was quite friable. We were able to dissect this out with Freer elevator. This came out quite nicely. The distal endpoint feathered off nicely, but we did place one single tacking suture at the 6-o'clock position. This was 7-0 Prolene. We then used the Impra carotid patch to close the arteriotomy site. This was done with a CV-7 Gore-Tex suture in a running fashion. We heparinized, backbled, and forebled. Intermittently, we had her move her left hand during the case. After suturing the suture line, we opened up the external carotid and the common carotid. After about 10 heartbeats, we then opened up the internal carotid artery. There was bleeding from needle holes. This was controlled with FloSeal. There was good flow through all the arteries at the end of the procedure by Doppler. A 10-mm flat Jackson-Pratt drain was placed before closure of the wound. Hemostasis was present. At the end of the procedure in the admit room, she was awake and following commands and moving all of her extremities. She went to the recovery room in stable condition. I met with the patient's family postoperatively to discuss the operation.

ADDENDUM: It should be noted that this procedure was done with intraoperative EEG monitoring. No changes were noted in the EEG during the procedure. Clamp time was 40 minutes. A patch closure was used as noted. She was also reversed with 40 mg of protamine at the end of the procedure.

28. OPERATIVE REPORT

INDICATION: Prolonged fetal heart rate deceleration. *(report delivery complicated by fetal heart rate)*

PROCEDURE: Vacuum-assisted vaginal delivery. *(report delivery vacuum assisted)*

Copyright © 2016 by Elsevier Inc.

COMPLICATIONS: Shoulder dystocia, relieved with McRobert's maneuver. *(report delivery complication due to shoulder presentation)*

PREAMBLE: The patient is a 33-year-old gravida 3, para 2, 38 week, 3 days gestation, admitted from the emergency department secondary to pelvic pain *(not reported because the pain is part of delivery)*. The patient was quite uncomfortable and had artificial rupture of membranes followed by labor progression to full dilation. She then began pushing, and some prolonged fetal heart rate decelerations down to about 90 beats per minute were noted *(supports delivery complicated by fetal heart rate)*. Because of this, a decision was made to proceed with vacuum extraction *(supports delivery vacuum assisted)* to assist in expediting delivery.

PROCEDURE NOTE: Maternal bladder was emptied using straight catheter. Pelvic examination was carried out and the cervix was confirmed to be fully dilated. Fetal vertex was present at +1 station. The small kiwi cup vacuum *(supports delivery vacuum assisted)* was then applied to the fetal vertex. On the second pull, there was one pop off but this was after good descent of the fetal head had been achieved. Baby then delivered and was a live-born male infant. *(report one liveborn with a V code)* There was moderate shoulder dystocia present *(supports delivery complicated by shoulder presentation)* and this was relieved with McRobert's maneuver. The baby was handed off to the NICU team and is currently in the NICU for further observation. Apgar's *(a newborn maturity scoring method)* are not available at this time. Cord blood gas is also pending. After an episiotomy, a second-degree perineal tear still occurred during delivery. *(for ICD-9-CM, report delivery complicated by second degree laceration of perineum with fifth digit "1" to indicate the complication occurred at the time of delivery)* This was repaired using 3-0 chromic in usual manner. The patient tolerated this procedure well. Estimated blood loss during delivery was 200 cc.

29. OPERATIVE REPORT

PREOPERATIVE DIAGNOSES:

1. Intrauterine pregnancy, 39 weeks.
2. Multiparity.
3. Desires permanent sterilization.
4. History of previous cesarean section × 2.

POSTOPERATIVE DIAGNOSES:

1. Intrauterine pregnancy, 39 weeks.
2. Multiparity.
3. Desires permanent sterilization.
4. History of previous cesarean section × 2.

PROCEDURE: Repeat low transverse cervical segment cesarean section with postpartum tubal ligation.

ANESTHESIA: Spinal.

ESTIMATED BLOOD LOSS: 800 cc

URINE OUTPUT: 40 cc

FLUIDS: 3000 cc

COMPLICATIONS: None.

Copyright © 2016 by Elsevier Inc.

FINDINGS: Viable male infant *(report the outcome of delivery)* weighing 6 pounds 10 ounces with Apgar's of 9 at 1 minute and 10 at 5 minutes.

PROCEDURE: The patient was prepped and draped in a supine position with left lateral displacement of the uterine fundus. Under spinal anesthesia and Foley catheter indwelling, a transverse incision was made in the lower abdomen using the old scar. The fascia was divided laterally. Rectus muscles were divided in the midline. The peritoneum was entered in a sharp manner. The incision was extended vertically. The bladder flap was created using sharp and blunt dissection and reflected inferiorly. The uterus was entered in a sharp manner in the lower uterine segment, and the incision was extended laterally with blunt traction. The head was delivered, the infant was delivered, and the infant was bulb suctioned while the cord was being doubly clamped and divided. The infant was given to the intensive care nursery staff in good condition. The placenta was manually expressed. Uterus was delivered through the abdominal cavity and placed on a wet lap sponge. A dry lap sponge was used to ensure that the remaining products of conception were removed. The cervical os was ensured patent with a ring forceps. The uterus incision was closed with 0 Vicryl in an interlocking suture in two layers with second layer imbricating the first. Figure-of-eight sutures were also placed as required for hemostasis. Operative site was inspected, irrigated, and hemostatic. The bladder flap was reapproximated using 2-0 Vicryl in a continuous suture in the midline. The left tube was identified in its entirety, including the fimbriated end and was grasped at its midportion and elevated. The mesosalpinx was transected using the Bovie. Approximately 3 cm of tube was isolated and excised. The proximal end of the distal portion and the distal end of the proximal portion were ligated with 0 chromic suture. The right tube was identified and ligated in the same fashion. Operative site was inspected and was hemostatic. Uterus was placed back in the midabdominal cavity. Pelvic gutters were irrigated. The anterior peritoneum was reapproximated with 2-0 Vicryl continuous suture. The incision was irrigated. Subcutaneous drain was placed, and the skin was closed with 2-0 silk. Sponges and needles were accounted for at the completion of the procedure. The patient left the operating room in apparent good condition after tolerating the procedure well. The Foley catheter was patent and draining a small amount of clear urine at the completion of the procedure.

30. OPERATIVE REPORT

PREOPERATIVE DIAGNOSIS: Complicated pregnancy with prior cesarean sections.

POSTOPERATIVE DIAGNOSIS: Complicated pregnancy with prior cesarean sections. *(Z/V code for history of obstetrical disorder affecting management of current pregnancy)*

PROCEDURE PERFORMED: Amniocentesis for fetal lung maturity. *(V code for screening, antenatal based on amniocentesis)*

INDICATIONS: The patient is at 38½-weeks' gestation and has had three prior C-sections and hospitalizations for recurrent episodes of pyelonephritis. *(Z/V code for personal history a specified urinary system disorder)* We desired to check fetal maturity so we could expedite delivery if possible.

Copyright © 2016 by Elsevier Inc.

PROCEDURE: The patient was scanned with ultrasound, and few pockets of amniotic fluid were noted; therefore, we elected to do a suprapubic tap. The abdomen was prepped and draped. Dr. Marco elevated the breech of the infant up out of the pelvis, and we scanned suprapubically and found a nice pocket of amniotic fluid. A single tap was done and 10 cc of clear yellow fluid obtained. This fluid was checked for pH and was deeply blue on Nitrazine, indicating it to be most likely amniotic fluid, not urine. She tolerated this well.

Cytology report later indicated slightly decreased fetal lung maturity based on levels of phosphatidylglycerol, with recommendation to re-evaluate in 10 days. *(abnormal amnion, affecting fetus)*

31. OPERATIVE REPORT

Colonoscopy and Polypectomy

PREOPERATIVE DIAGNOSIS: Hematochezia.

POSTOPERATIVE DIAGNOSIS: Two small polyps in the cecum ascending colon, hot biopsied off. A small rectal polyp, hot biopsied off.

INDICATION: This is a 46-year-old white male with Tourette's and some MR who has had some hematochezia. There are no risk factors with no other symptoms.

PREOPERATIVE MEDICATIONS: Fentanyl 100 mcg IV; Versed 4 mg IV.

FINDINGS: The Pentax video colonoscope was inserted without difficulty to the cecum. The ileocecal valve was identified. The appendiceal orifice was seen. I could not enter the cecum. Just above the valve, there was a small 2- to 3-cm polyp. This was hot biopsied off. There was a sessile 3-mm polyp in the proximal ascending colon, hot biopsied off. Inspection of the remainder of the ascending colon, hepatic flexure, transverse colon, splenic flexure, descending colon, and sigmoid colon, revealed no erythema, ulceration, exudate, friability, or other mucosal abnormalities. The rectum showed a small 2-mm polyp that was hot biopsied off. The patient tolerated the procedure well.

IMPRESSION: Three small polyps, two in the cecum ascending colon area and one on the rectum, hot biopsied off.

PLAN: If these polyps are adenomatous, the patient should return again in 5 years for surveillance.

PATHOLOGY REPORT LATER INDICATED: See Report 56.

32. OPERATIVE REPORT

PREOPERATIVE DIAGNOSIS: Nonhealing duodenal ulcer.

POSTOPERATIVE DIAGNOSIS: Nonhealing duodenal ulcer.

PROCEDURES PERFORMED:

1. Exploratory laparotomy.
2. Partial gastrectomy (antrectomy).
3. Truncal vagotomy.
4. Gastrojejunostomy.
5. Cholecystectomy with intraoperative cholangiogram.

Copyright © 2016 by Elsevier Inc.

INDICATION: The patient is a 60-year-old female who presented with a nonhealing gastric ulcer. She has had symptoms for about a year. She complains of epigastric pain. Medical therapy with Prilosec failed, as did therapy for *H. pylori*. Biopsy of the ulcer has been done, and it was benign. The patient had a negative workup for gastrinoma. Calcium level was also normal. The patient now presents for exploratory laparotomy and partial gastrectomy. The risks and benefits were discussed with the patient in detail. She understood and agreed to proceed.

PROCEDURE: The patient was brought to the operating room. Her abdomen was prepped and draped in a sterile fashion. A midline umbilical incision was made. The peritoneal cavity was entered. Initial inspection of the peritoneal cavity showed normal liver, spleen, colon, and small bowel. There was an ulcer along the first portion of the duodenum just beyond the pylorus with some scarring. There was also an ulcer in the posterior part of the duodenal bulb, which was penetrating to the pancreas. We started dissection along the greater curvature of the stomach. Vessels were ligated with 2-0 silk ties. There was an enlarged lymph node along the greater curvature of the stomach, which was sent for frozen section. It proved to be a benign lymph node. This was the only enlarged node found during dissection. We then proceeded with truncal vagotomy. The anterior vagus and posterior vagus were identified. They were clipped proximally and distally, and a segment of each nerve was excised and sent for frozen section, and a segment of both vagus nerves was excised and confirmed by frozen section. An incision was made around the gastrohepatic ligament. The mesentery along the lesser curvature of the stomach was dissected. The vessels were ligated with 2-0 silk ties along the lesser curvature of the stomach. A Kocher maneuver was performed to aid mobilization. The pancreas was completely normal. No masses were found in the pancreas. There was penetration of the ulcer in the superior part of the head of the pancreas. Dissection was continued posterior to the stomach. The adhesions posterior to the stomach were taken down. The ulcer was in the posterior segment of the duodenal bulb just beyond the pylorus and it had penetrated the pancreas. All the posterior layer of the ulcer that was left adherent to the pancreas was shaved off. The stomach was divided with the GIA stapler so that the complete antrum would be in the specimen. The duodenum was divided between clamps. The stomach pylorus and first part of the duodenum were sent to pathology for examination. Then the duodenal stump was closed with running suture. Using 3-0 Lembert sutures, the posterior wall of the ulcer was incorporated for duodenal closure. The base of the duodenum was rolled over the ulcer, and it was all-incorporating to the duodenal closure. Our next step was to proceed with cholecystectomy. The gallbladder was separated from the liver, reflected, and taken down, and the gallbladder was divided from the liver with blunt dissection and cautery. The cystic artery was doubly ligated with silk. The cystic duct was identified. The cystic duct and gallbladder junction and gallbladder ducts were identified. Intraoperative cholangiogram was performed showing free flow of bile into the intrahepatic duct and into the duodenum. No leaks were seen. The cystic duct was doubly ligated, and the gallbladder was sent to pathology. The staple line in the proximal stomach was oversewn with 3-0 silk Lembert sutures. A retrocolic isoperistaltic Hofmeister-type gastrojejunostomy was performed on the remaining stomach and loop of jejunum. This was an isoperistaltic end-to-side two-layer anastomosis with 3-0 chromic and 3-0 silk. The stomach was secured to the transverse mesocolon with several interrupted silk sutures to prevent any herniation along the retrocolic space.

Copyright © 2016 by Elsevier Inc.

The anastomosis had a good lumen and good blood supply. There was no twist along the anastomosis. Before the anastomosis was finished, a nasogastric tube was placed along the afferent limb of the jejunum to decompress the duodenum and prevent blow out of the duodenal stump. Extra holes were made in the NG tube to provide adequate drainage. The anastomosis was marked with two clips on each side, and a Jackson-Pratt drain was placed over the duodenal stump. The peritoneal cavity was irrigated until clear. Hemostasis was adequate. The fascia was then closed with interrupted 0 Ethibond sutures. Skin edges were approximated with staples. Subcutaneous tissues were irrigated before closure. Estimated blood loss throughout the procedure was 200 ml. IV fluids: 3400 ml. Urine output: 840 ml.

FINDINGS:
1. Nonhealing benign ulcer in the posterior duodenal bulb penetrating into the head of the pancreas.
2. Partial gastrectomy *(antrectomy performed)* and excision of the pylorus, first portion of the duodenum along with ulcer.
3. Hofmeister-type retrocolic isoperistaltic gastrojejunostomy.
4. Posterior wall of the ulcer that was penetrating into the pancreas incorporated into closure of the duodenal stump.
5. Truncal vagotomy performed with intraoperative frozen section confirming both vagus nerves.
6. Cholecystectomy performed due to chronic cholecystitis with normal intraoperative cholangiogram.
7. Jackson-Pratt drain placed over the duodenal stump.

The items that are to be coded are listed below:

Partial gastrectomy *(antrectomy)* with gastrojejunostomy
Truncal vagotomy
Cholecystectomy with intraoperative cholangiogram

PATHOLOGY REPORT LATER INDICATED: Tissue showed no evidence of carcinoma. The radiologist reported the x-ray with 74300.

33. OPERATIVE REPORT

PREOPERATIVE DIAGNOSIS: Fournier's gangrene.

POSTOPERATIVE DIAGNOSIS: Fournier's gangrene, gastric foreign bodies.

PROCEDURES PERFORMED:

1. Exploratory laparotomy with gastrotomy and removal of gastric foreign body.
2. Placement of 18-French Moss gastrojejunostomy feeding tube.
3. Diverting end-sigmoid colostomy *(Hartmann's procedure)*.

ANESTHESIA: General.

INDICATIONS: This is a 33-year-old patient with Fournier's gangrene who presents today for a diverting colostomy due to wound care and placement of a gastrostomy tube for help with further follow-up feeding. He presents today for exploration. The family understands the risks of bleeding, infection, and postoperative fluid collections and wishes to proceed.

Copyright © 2016 by Elsevier Inc.

PROCEDURE: The patient was brought to the operating room, placed under general anesthesia, and prepped and draped with Betadine solution. A midline incision was made with a #10 blade and dissection was carried down through subcutaneous tissues using electrocautery. The midline fascia was identified and divided. The posterior sheath and peritoneum were sharply incised, thus allowing entry into the peritoneal cavity. There was some free fluid within the peritoneal cavity but no evidence of any abnormalities. We first identified the stomach and could feel what we felt were some polyps in the stomach. We first placed concentric purse-string sutures along the greater curvature of the stomach, opened up the stomach, and then passed an 18-French Moss gastrojejunostomy tube but were unable to get it down through the pylorus. We could feel these multiple masses in the stomach. We tied the purse-string sutures and inflated the balloon. We then made a small opening in the stomach with electrocautery and retrieved about 20 large what appeared to be vegetable matter and partially digested peppers and pickles. We irrigated with saline and then were able to pass the Moss gastrojejunostomy tube, the distal end, down through the pylorus. We closed the gastrotomy with a running 3-0 Vicryl and an outer layer of 3-0 silk Lembert sutures. We irrigated this area well. We then identified the sigmoid colon, fired a TLC-75 stapler across the sigmoid/ descending colon, and then placed a 3-0 Prolene on the rectal stump. We divided the mesentery between right angle clamps and tied the pedicles with 3-0 silk ties. We had a previously marked stomal opening in the left lower quadrant. We grasped this with a Kocher clamp, made an elliptical incision around this, and then divided the anterior sheath of the rectus in cruciate fashion, divided through the rectus muscles, and then opened the posterior sheath and peritoneum. We brought the colon then through this area. There was good mobility of the colon, and the colon was viable. We then irrigated the abdomen with saline, and, once all sponge and needle counts were correct, we closed the midline fascia with a combination of interrupted 0 Vicryl and running 0 PDS. The skin was closed with skin clips. The staple line was then removed from the colon and the colostomy was matured with 3-0 Vicryl sutures. An appliance was placed. All sponge and needle counts were correct. He tolerated this well.

Prior to leaving the operating room, we took down the dressings of his right leg. There was good granulation tissue, which was pink and viable, and we then re-dressed the wound and sent him back to the surgical critical care unit in critical but stable condition.

PATHOLOGY REPORT LATER INDICATED: Idiopathic gangrene. Numerous undigested vegetable matter.

34. OPERATIVE REPORT

PREOPERATIVE DIAGNOSIS: Severe internal and external hemorrhoids.

POSTOPERATIVE DIAGNOSIS: Same.

PROCEDURE PERFORMED: Three quadrant hemorrhoidectomy.

ANESTHESIA: Spinal.

INDICATION: This is a very pleasant female who presents today with severe internal and external hemorrhoids for elective excision. She understands the risks of bleeding, infection, and postoperative fluid collection. She wishes to proceed.

Copyright © 2016 by Elsevier Inc.

PROCEDURE: The patient was brought to the operating room and placed under spinal anesthesia, prepped, and draped sterilely with Betadine solution. Digital rectal examination was first performed. There were severe external hemorrhoids. Pratt anoscope was inserted. The severest of the hemorrhoids were at the 6-o'clock, 9-o'clock, and 3-o'clock positions. These were each grasped with an Allis clamp, excised in diamond shape fashion. The mucosal defects were closed with running locked 3-0 Vicryl with the suture lines imbricated with 3-0 chromic sutures. This gave us a good closure that was hemostatic. We anesthetized the area with 30 cc of 0.5% Sensorcaine with epinephrine solution and then placed four gauze in the rectal canal. She tolerated this well and was taken to recovery in stable condition.

PATHOLOGY REPORT LATER INDICATED: Benign tissue.

35. OPERATIVE REPORT

PROCEDURE: Placement of CORFLO, feeding tube.

INDICATION: Feeding, patient with gastroparesis.

PROCEDURE: The patient was placed in the sitting position and then tilted to the right with a wedge. CORFLO was placed at the level of 19 cm without any complications. KUB was then done demonstrating the tip of the CORFLO in the third portion of the duodenum. After confirmation of postpyloric position of the CORFLO, the patient was started on Ultracal at 10 cc/hr.

36. OPERATIVE REPORT

PREOPERATIVE DIAGNOSES:

1. Expressed desire of the operating gynecologist to insert indwelling ureteral stents for ease of dissection of the anticipated enlarged adherent uterus.
2. Gynecologic diagnosis of pelvic endometriosis.

POSTOPERATIVE DIAGNOSES: Same.

PROCEDURE PERFORMED: Cystourethroscopy, insertion of bilateral ureteral catheters.

PROCEDURE: After general anesthesia and after the abdomen and genitalia had been prepped and draped in the usual fashion, the patient was placed in the dorsolithotomy position. The genitalia were examined and proved to be essentially unremarkable. The urethra was instrumented with a 24-French panendoscope sheath, and, using the foroblique and right-angle lenses, inspection of the entire vesical cavity showed no indication of any pathologic lesion. There is slight indention and some of the bladder incident to the uterine impression. The two ureteral orifices appear to be essentially unremarkable. The left ureteral orifice was catheterized with a 6-French Whistle Tip catheter with ease. The catheter was advanced to approximately 25 cm on the left side. Attention was then directed to the right side, and the right ureteral orifice was catheterized with a 6-French Whistle Tip catheter. The catheter was placed at approximately 24 cm. The bladder was then entered, Panendoscope sheath was withdrawn. A 18-French 5-ml balloon Foley catheter was then inserted into the bladder and left indwelling to the Foley catheter. The two ureteral catheters were

Copyright © 2016 by Elsevier Inc.

anchored with no. 1 black silk. The two ureteral catheters and the Foley catheters were then connected to straight drainage and the patient was removed from the dorsolithotomy position. Dr. Weasly, the patient's gynecologist, then proceeded with a total abdominal hysterectomy and bilateral salpingo-oophorectomy.

37. OPERATIVE REPORT

PREOPERATIVE DIAGNOSIS: Recurrent transitional cell carcinoma of the bladder.

POSTOPERATIVE DIAGNOSIS: Same.

PROCEDURE PERFORMED: Cystoscopy; multiple random bladder biopsies.

CLINICAL NOTE: This patient has recurrent transitional cell carcinoma of the bladder. He has had BCG bladder instillation to help prevent recurrence. His last instillation was 6 weeks ago. The patient is doing well. He denied any complaints.

PROCEDURE: The patient was given a general endotracheal anesthetic and prepped and draped in lithotomy position. A 24-French resectoscope was passed into the bladder under direct vision. The urethra was normal. Prostate was nonobstructed. Inspection of the bladder demonstrated areas of hyperemia that would be most consistent with BCG changes but might also represent recurrent TCC. These areas were biopsied using a cold-cup biopsy. A 24-French resectoscope loupe was then used to cauterize these areas. Ureteric orifices were identified. Clear urine could be seen effluxing bilaterally.

The patient tolerated the procedure well. A B&O suppository was placed rectally after the end of the procedure. An 18-French Foley catheter was placed to straight drainage. Bimanual examination showed no significant abnormality and the prostate felt normal.

The patient will be scheduled for recheck cystoscopy in three months time providing pathology shows no evidence of recurrent tumor.

ADDENDUM: Total resected and fulgurated area of the bladder was 7 square centimeters.

PATHOLOGY REPORT LATER INDICATED: See Report 55.

38. OPERATIVE REPORT

PREOPERATIVE DIAGNOSIS: Urinary incontinence.

POSTOPERATIVE DIAGNOSIS: Same.

PROCEDURE PERFORMED: Insertion of double cuff artificial urinary sphincter with 25 cc reservoir (multicomponent).

CLINICAL NOTE: This patient has had radiation for prostate cancer. This recurred. He then had cryotherapy. His PSA is undetectable but he has significant urinary incontinence unresponsive to pharmacotherapy. External clamp devices have been unsatisfactory.

PROCEDURE NOTE: The patient was given a spinal anesthetic, prepped and draped in a supine position. A penoscrotal incision was made. A 16-French Foley was placed in the bladder to straight drainage. The urethra was

Copyright © 2016 by Elsevier Inc.

dissected to the level of the bulb. The bulbocavernous muscle was very atrophic and was not dissected off the urethra. A double cuff placement was selected. The urethra was mobilized in two places with a small bridge of tissue between them. These cuffs were incised. Both were incised at 4.5 cm. A reservoir space was created by manual dissection in the left inguinal canal into the retropubic space. The reservoir was placed, cycled, and filled with 25 cc of sterile saline. Both cuffs were placed in the usual fashion. The pump was then placed in the mid-scrotal pouch. Connections were made using a Y connector and straight connectors in the usual fashion. The system was cycled; it worked well. Foley catheter was withdrawn to insure cycling appropriately. Subcutaneous tissues were closed with 3-0 chromic and skin with a 4-0 subcuticular Vicryl stitch. The pump was cycled again and then deactivated; the Foley catheter replaced. The patient tolerated the procedure well and was transferred to the recovery room in good condition. The wounds were thoroughly irrigated with Bacitracin solution.

39. OPERATIVE REPORT

PREOPERATIVE DIAGNOSIS: Morbid obesity.

POSTOPERATIVE DIAGNOSIS: Same.

PROCEDURES:

1. Laparoscopic Roux-en-Y gastrointestinal bypass.
2. Liver biopsy.

ANESTHESIA: General.

INDICATION: The patient is a 36-year-old female who presents with morbid obesity, with a current BMI of 46.0. She has gone to the seminars, and we have discussed laparoscopic Roux-en-Y gastrointestinal bypass along with the risk of surgery including bleeding, infection, leakage from the anastomoses, conversion to open procedure, postoperative stenoses of the anastomoses, or bowel obstruction. She understands and wishes to proceed.

PROCEDURE: The patient was brought to the operating room and placed under general anesthesia. A Foley catheter and orogastric tubes were inserted. She was prepped and draped sterilely with Betadine solution. A supraumbilical incision was made with a #15 blade, and dissection was carried down through the subcutaneous tissues bluntly. The patient had an incisional hernia from an old trocar port site. We placed our operative trocar into the abdomen, insufflated the abdomen. There was no damage to the underlying viscera. Under direct vision, we then placed two, midclavicular line, 12-millimeter ports that were just lateral and above the umbilical port. There was a right upper quadrant 12-millimeter port in the anterior axillary line and a left upper quadrant 5-millimeter port in the anterior axillary line. These were all placed under direct vision with no damage to the bowel. The patient had some adhesions of her gastrohepatic ligament to the liver. We took these down using the harmonic scalpel. Before continuing, a needle specimen was obtained from the liver, appropriately marked for pathologic evaluation. We then entered the retrogastric space and placed our taut catheter behind the stomach. We then flipped the omentum up over the top of itself. We elevated the transverse colon and opened the transverse colon where we could see the drain. We identified the ligament of Treitz and fired an Endo-GIA stapler across the bowel, down from the ligament of Treitz. We fired an additional load across the mesentery. We then counted

Copyright © 2016 by Elsevier Inc.

out 100 centimeters of bowel and then performed a stapled side-to-side functional end-to-end anastomosis by opening the bowel on the proximal and distal sides with the harmonic scalpel, firing two loads of the Endo-GIA stapler and closing the anastomosis with an Endo-GIA fired staple line. This gave us a nice anastomosis. We closed the mesenteric defect here with an Ethibond suture and fixed with Laparoties. We then sutured the proximal end to the catheter and flipped the mesentery back down. We then brought the bowel and the catheter up in retrogastric fashion. Next, we identified the angle of His. We opened the angle of His, and we fired five loads of the Endo-GIA stapler across the stomach. We had blown up the 20-cc balloon and had about a 20-cc pouch. Once we had completely transected the stomach, we went above and placed the Bioenteric catheter within the gastric pouch. We passed the snare through it. We made a separate stab incision in the upper abdomen and passed the wire through. We then fed the anvil end of the CEA-21 stapler down through the back of the pharynx down through the esophagus and brought out through our gastric pouch. We then enlarged the left midclavicular line, abdominal port, and placed the CEA-25 stapler through here. We opened the staple line on the bowel that we had brought up after we had removed the taut catheter and placed the CEA stapler into the bowel, brought the spike through, connected the two ends of the CEA, closed it, and fired it. This gave us a nice 21-millimeter circular anastomosis. We completed the anastomosis with the Endo-GIA stapler. We imbricated the staple line with two Ethibond sutures, placed a wad of fat over the last to adhere the fat near our staple line. We tested the anastomosis with air with the bowel clamped, and there was no evidence of a leak. We then placed Hemaseel over this anastomosis, and then once again mobilized the mesentery. We then closed the mesenteric defect where the small bowel had gone in retrogastric fashion with the Ethicon Endo-suture. We once again placed Hemaseel on our small anastomosis. We placed 10 flat Jackson-Pratt drains near our GJ anastomosis, which came on out the left side. We removed the trocar ports under direct vision. We then extended our umbilical incision and reduced the umbilical hernia. We closed the fascial defect with interrupted 0 Prolene sutures. We anesthetized the wounds at all areas with a total of 60 cc of 0.50% Sensorcaine with epinephrine solution. We secured the drains in place with 0 silk sutures and then closed the skin with 3-0 Prolene sutures. Steri-Strips and sterile Band-Aids were applied. All sponge and needle counts were correct. We left the taut catheter and a Penrose drain in the left midclavicular line incision.

All sponge and needle counts were correct. She tolerated this well and was taken to recovery in stable condition.

PATHOLOGY REPORT LATER INDICATED: See Report 63.

40. OPERATIVE REPORT

HISTORY: This patient, who is unknown to me, reports working in the shop at his home grinding metal approximately 5 hours ago. He was wearing safety glasses, but he has noticed a foreign body in his right eye. He reports slight irritation to the eye. Denies blurred vision.

PHYSICAL EXAMINATION: PERLA, fundi without edema. There was no foreign body on lid eversion. Slit lamp shows a foreign body approximately 2 to 3 o'clock on the edge of the cornea. This foreign body appears metallic. There is very small area of rust around the site. Iris is intact. There are no cells in the anterior chamber. Fluorescein dye reveals uptake only over foreign body.

Copyright © 2016 by Elsevier Inc.

PROCEDURE: Two drops of Alcaine were used in the right eye. Foreign body was removed with an eye spud without difficulty. Slight orange discoloration at the base of cornea, but no definite rust ring visible.

IMPRESSION: Residual corneal abrasion.

DISPOSITION: Foreign body removed from right eye.

41. OPERATIVE REPORT

PREOPERATIVE DIAGNOSIS: Left cervical spondylosis, C5–6, C6–7, with cervical discs.

POSTOPERATIVE DIAGNOSIS: Same.

PROCEDURE PERFORMED: Anterior discectomy and osteophytectomy for decompression at C5–6 and C6–7, with allograft fusion and Zephyr plating.
   This case was monitored with sensory evoked potentials throughout the case. There were no changes.

PROCEDURE: Under general anesthesia, the patient was placed in the cervical outrigger. The neck was prepped and draped in the usual manner. An incision was made parallel to the sternocleidomastoid, and then we got onto the omohyoid and incised this. Then with sharp dissection we got onto the prevertebral fascia, put the Farley-Thompson retractor in, and then I was able to localize the C5–6 and C6–7 interspaces. The plan here was to decompress the nerve roots and get rid of the ridges, the disc, and to fuse and plate. The discectomies were done at C5–6 and C6–7. The ridges were removed, the discs were removed, and then the cartilaginous surfaces were prepared for reception of the bony fusion. At C6–7, a #8 trial was utilized and at C5–6 a #7 trial was utilized with bone. I took off the ridges, I took off the osteophytes, I removed the discs. I got down to the dura on both sides and was satisfied now that the nerve roots were decompressed and I could put the trial in and place the structural bone graft in. This was done at both levels. This having been done, they were countersunk and I then utilized a Zephyr plate from C5 down to C7 and put a screw into C6 as well. This done, a Hemovac drain was placed into the wound. Of course, the plate was locked, and we then closed the wound in layers utilizing 2-0 chromic on the platysma with 2-0 plain in the subcutaneous tissue and 3-0 nylon interrupted mattress sutures on the skin. A dressing was applied. The patient was to wear a collar in the postop period.

PATHOLOGY REPORT LATER INDICATED: Benign bone and tissue.

42. OPERATIVE REPORT

PREOPERATIVE DIAGNOSES:

1. Ptosis, right upper lid.
2. Loss of superior visual field secondary to #1.
3. Superior hemianopia secondary to #1, right eye.

POSTOPERATIVE DIAGNOSES: Same.

PROCEDURE PERFORMED: Fasanella-Servat procedure, right upper lid.

Copyright © 2016 by Elsevier Inc.

ANESTHESIA: General endotracheal.

INDICATIONS: This 57-year-old white female has had progressively drooping lid on her right for many years which has now reduced her superior visual field in the right eye and has actually limited her vision. After the prior approval and the photos and documentation were obtained, it was noted that the patient did have a 3- to 4-mm ptosis of the right upper lid and we would approach this with a Fasanella-Servat procedure. The risk of infection, hemorrhage and reoperations were discussed.

PROCEDURE: After the patient was placed under suitable general endotracheal anesthesia; the superior tarsal border was then marked with a marking pen and a 15 Bard-Parker blade cut down through skin to the muscle area. The lid was then everted on a Desmarres retractor and two curved mosquitos were then placed with the point central and pointing superiorly when the lid was everted. A 6-0 gut rapid absorbing suture was then started through the skin incision at the superior tarsal border and then a purse string was then woven along the curve tips and then the 3 to 4 mm resection was then obtained and then the serpentine 6-0 gut suture was then approximated without cutting it and brought out through the skin and tied. It was allowed to retract into the knot. There was no bleeding and there was no cut suture. Maxitrol ointment, a Telfa pad, and patch was applied and the patient was sent to the recovery room. There were no complications.

43. OPERATIVE REPORT

PREOPERATIVE DIAGNOSIS: Lumbar radiculopathy secondary to herniated L5-S1 disc.

POSTOPERATIVE DIAGNOSIS: Same.

PROCEDURE PERFORMED: Right L5-S1 hemilaminectomy with excision of herniated L5-S1 disc.

PROCEDURE: The patient was taken to the operating room and placed under general endotracheal anesthesia. He was rotated into the prone position on chest rolls with arms extended over the head. The lumbar region was shaved, prepped, and draped in the usual sterile manner. The proposed vertical midline incision was infiltrated with lidocaine, with epinephrine. The skin was incised and sharp dissection carried through the subcutaneous tissues. The fascia was incised and subperiosteal dissection undertaken at L5-S1. The hemilamina of L5 was then removed in piecemeal fashion. This allowed evaluation of both the L4–5 disc as well as the L5-S1 disc. At L5-S1, moderate-sized disc herniation was immediately evident. The surrounding capsule was incised, and a large fragment of ligamentous degenerative disc was removed. The interspace was then probed, and all degenerative disc material was removed. On completion, the thecal sac and nerve root were noted to be well decompressed at L4–5. The L4–5 level appeared normal. Epidural space was lined with Surgicel and fat graft, and the wound closed in interrupted layers, with 4-0 Vicryl subcuticular stitch for skin. Steri-Strips and sterile dressing were applied to the wound. The patient tolerated the procedure well and was transferred to the recovery room in good condition.

PATHOLOGY REPORT LATER INDICATED: See Report 57.

Copyright © 2016 by Elsevier Inc.

44. OPERATIVE REPORT

PREOPERATIVE DIAGNOSES:

1. Left orbitonasal mass.
2. Dry eye syndrome.
3. Pseudophakia, both eyes.
4. Computerized tomography confirmed tumor left orbital, left nasal side.

POSTOPERATIVE DIAGNOSES: Same with the addition of low-grade lymphoma, left orbit.

PROCEDURE: Anterior orbitotomy, debulking and biopsy.

ANESTHESIA: General endotracheal anesthesia.

INDICATION: This 81-year-old white woman has had a progressively enlarging mass of the left superior nasal orbit, which had become quite hard and is attached to the bone. CT shows there has been no bony invasion, and the brain has not been invaded. More than likely, this is a lymphoma, but we want to take the patient for an anterior orbitotomy for debulking and biopsy.

DESCRIPTION OF PROCEDURE: After the patient was prepped and draped in the usual sterile fashion for ophthalmic surgery, the superior sulcus fold was marked out on her medial left upper lid. This was then cut through skin and muscle with the 25 Bard-Parker blade down through the orbital fat pad. It was noted there was some saponified fat and a hard mass that was kind of an orangish-red color and was attached to this. Two specimens were removed and tagged and sent for frozen section, and into the cryo unit with liquid nitrogen down to −80 degrees and was then brought in to remove the rest of the mass. There were some fragments of mass still attached to the nasal wall of the orbit. The frozen section revealed lymphoma, low grade, probably stage I, and since this is radiosensitive and that all of the tumor could not be removed without exenterating the orbit, it was elected to close at this point and treat the rest conservatively. The wound was closed after the remaining tumor was infiltrated with Solu-Medrol 125 mg per ml for a total of 2 ml, after which the wound was closed with interrupted 6-0 black nylon suture and Maxitrol ointment. Telfa pad, patch and shield were applied. The patient was sent to the recovery room. There were no complications.

PATHOLOGY REPORT LATER INDICATED: Lymphoma.

45. RADIOLOGY REPORT

EXAMINATION OF: Chest.

CLINICAL SYMPTOMS: Chest pain.

PORTABLE CHEST, AP SITTING (ONE VIEW), 4:45 PM: Comparisons are made with the previous study of 08/23/XX. The cardiac silhouette is not grossly enlarged for this projection. The mediastinum is not widened. Lung fields are generally clear and expanded to the periphery. Cardiac monitors do superimpose the chest.

CONCLUSION: Generally stable appearance of the chest, unchanged compared with the previous study.

Copyright © 2016 by Elsevier Inc.

46. RADIOLOGY REPORT

EXAMINATION OF: Biophysical profile.

CLINICAL SYMPTOMS: High blood pressure, estimated gestational age 28 weeks 5 days.

BIOPHYSICAL PROFILE: The placenta is located along the anterior wall. It is heterogeneous in echotexture, grade II. The AFI is 5.4 cm, which is low. Fetal motion noted by the technologist. Heart rate 147 beats per minute. Intrauterine hypoechoic area seen anteriorly within the uterus measures about 2 cm in size and a second similar sized hypoechoic area is located within the uterus. Both findings are presumed fibroids.

They are nonspecific findings, however. Biophysical profile was scored a perfect 8 out of 8.

47. CT SCAN

EXAMINATION OF: CT of orbits.

CLINICAL SYMPTOMS: Left eye pain.

CT OF ORBITS: CT of orbits in axial and coronal planes without contrast. Patient was vomiting therefore contrast was not given.

1. Complete opacification of right aspect of sphenoid sinus.
2. Near complete opacification of right maxillary antrum.
3. Polypoid membrane thickening left maxillary antrum.
4. Scattered membrane thickening throughout a few ethmoidal air cells.
5. Remainder negative.

48. MRA REPORT

EXAMINATION OF: MRA brain.

CLINICAL SYMPTOMS: Third nerve palsy, complete.

MAGNETIC RESONANCE EXAMINATION OF THE ARTERIAL VASCULATURE OF THE POSTERIOR FOSSA AND CIRCLE OF WILLIS REGION was performed utilizing three-dimensional time-of-flight multislab technique. Raw data and selected maximum-intensity projection images were photographed. Additionally, I have personally manipulated the maximum-intensity projections on a computer console in order to view the vasculature from various angulations.

I don't appreciate evidence of aneurysm. In particular, I don't appreciate evidence of aneurysm in the region of the posterior communicating arteries. I have personally reviewed the raw data images.

Bilaterally, there is some signal loss at the origin of the A1 segment of each anterior cerebral artery. This gives the appearance of stenosis. Most probably, this is technical, rather than due to true stenosis, but stenosis is not ruled out.

Internal carotid arteries appear unremarkable. Vertebral arteries are unremarkable. The basilar artery is unremarkable.

Proximal segments of the middle and posterior cerebral arteries appear unremarkable. Posterior communicating arteries are not visualized and are most probably very small.

Copyright © 2016 by Elsevier Inc.

49. RADIOLOGY REPORT

EXAMINATION OF: X-Ray Abdomen; single view.

CLINICAL SYMPTOMS: Malnutrition.

FINDINGS: A single supine view of the abdomen is submitted for interpretation. The majority of the pelvis and a portion of the left side of the abdomen are excluded from this examination. Feeding tube is identified. The tip overlies the left upper quadrant. Air is present within both small and large bowel, which does not appear distended as visualized on this examination. There is degenerative change and dextroscoliosis of the lumbar spine. Surgical clips overlie the right upper quadrant. Opacity is noted in the left lung base, which may relate to atelectasis or infiltrate. Follow-up is suggested.

50. RADIOLOGY REPORT

EXAMINATION OF: Left foot.

CLINICAL SYMPTOMS: Severe foot pain.

TWO VIEWS, LEFT FOOT: Comparison is made with the most recent films available 10/15/XX. There is diffuse demineralization of the osseous structures of the foot. Soft-tissue swelling is seen. Erosive changes have been previously described involving multiple metatarsophalangeal joints, and these are identified once again today. The differential is not significantly changed compared with the previous examination.

IMPRESSION:

1. Overall there is no significant interval change compared with 10/15/XX. There are extensive demineralization and extensive erosive changes involving the metatarsophalangeal joints and digits as described previously. Large cystic lesion is identified within the calcaneus as previously seen.
2. Diffuse soft-tissue swelling and inferior calcaneal spur.

51. CT REPORT

CT of Abdomen

CLINICAL HISTORY: Increased liver enzyme.

TECHNIQUE: The patient was scanned from the dome of the diaphragm through the iliac crest after administration of oral and intravenous contrast.

COMPARISON: Comparison is made with a previous ultrasound examination dated 11/18/XX.

FINDINGS: Evaluation of the liver demonstrates mildly decreased attenuation to be present throughout the liver diffusely. No focal abnormalities are present within the liver. The spleen, pancreas, kidneys, and adrenal glands appear unremarkable. No enlarged lymph nodes are seen within the abdomen. No abnormal fluid collections are seen within the abdomen. The lung bases appear clear. No pleural effusions are seen.

Copyright © 2016 by Elsevier Inc.

IMPRESSION:

1. There is diffusely decreased attenuation present within the liver. This suggests the presence of fatty infiltration of the liver. No focal abnormalities are seen within the liver.
2. The remainder of the CT examination of the abdomen appears unremarkable.

52. LUNG SCAN REPORT

EXAMINATION OF: Ventilation-perfusion lung scan.

CLINICAL SYMPTOMS: Shortness of breath.

VENTILATION-PERFUSION LUNG SCAN:

DOSE: 2.0 millicuries of technetium-99m DTPA via aerosol. 6.0 millicuries of technetium-99m MAA IV. Comparison is made with chest radiograph obtained at the same time.

There is inhomogeneity regarding ventilatory scan. This is seen bilaterally. There appears to be elevation of the right hemidiaphragm.

There is decreased perfusion and ventilation along the right posterior lung base. The patient is noted to have pulmonary opacities and pleural effusions on chest radiograph. Small area of decreased perfusion and ventilation noted along the posterior aspect of the left upper lobe. Overall findings indeterminate for pulmonary embolus.

IMPRESSION: Indeterminate probability for pulmonary embolus.

53. MRI REPORT

EXAMINATION OF: Myocardial perfusion imaging.

CLINICAL SYMPTOMS: Chest pain, shortness of breath.

MYOCARDIAL PERFUSION IMAGING: CARDIOLITE HEART IMAGING: SPECT left ventricular myocardial perfusion imaging study was performed in this patient. 29.5 millicuries of technetium-99m sestamibi was injected intravenously at peak stress. The patient had a maximal heart rate of 88%.

Evaluation of the qualitative image series shows the left ventricular myocardium to have a normal uptake of tracer. There is no evidence to suggest myocardial infarction or stress-induced ischemia.

IMPRESSION: Normal Cardiolite heart imaging as described above.

54. FROM OPERATIVE REPORT 20

CLINICAL HISTORY: C/C clear cell CA pelvis.

SPECIMEN RECEIVED: A. Endocervical curettings. B. Endometrial biopsy.

GROSS DESCRIPTION:

A. The specimen is labeled with the patient's name and "ecc" and consists of specimen jar with negligible tissue. The specimen is filtered and placed in one cassette.
B. The specimen is labeled with the patient's name and "endometrial" and consists of approximately 1 cc of wispy fragments.

Copyright © 2016 by Elsevier Inc.

MICROSCOPIC DESCRIPTION:

A. Sections show no tissue after processing.

Sections show fragments of tissue consisting predominantly of endocervical tissue and lower uterine segment. The endometrial glands are lined by 1 to 2 layers of columnar epithelium. Malignant clear cell carcinoma is microscopically identified.

DIAGNOSIS:

A. Endocervical curettings: Malignant clear cell carcinoma identified.

Endometrial biopsy: Scant fragments of endocervical mucosa and lower uterine segment; Grade 3, secondary, malignant endocervix and endometrium clear cell carcinoma, Primary site unknown.

55. FROM OPERATIVE REPORT 37

CLINICAL HISTORY: Bladder cancer.

SPECIMEN RECEIVED: Random bladder biopsy.

GROSS DESCRIPTION: The specimen is labeled with "biopsy" and consists of 3 specimens processed in toto, and random bladder pink-tan tissue biopsies in 1 cassette.

MICROSCOPIC DESCRIPTION: Sections show fragments of bladder mucosa showing vascularization and congestion with mild lymphocytic, plasma cell infiltrates, and lymphoid aggregates. The urothelium varies from normal to moderate to severe dysplasia to carcinoma in situ with full-thickness cytologic atypia and occasional mitoses. One fragment shows grade 2 papillary transitional cell carcinoma. The underlying lamina propria shows reactive fibroblasts with scattered lymphocytic, plasma cell, and eosinophilic infiltrates with admixed multinucleated giant cells. No definitive stromal invasion is identified.

DIAGNOSIS: Random bladder biopsies: Moderate to severe urothelial dysplasia/transitional cell carcinoma in situ and noninvasive grade 2 *(of 3)* papillary transitional cell carcinoma.

56. FROM OPERATIVE REPORT 31

CLINICAL HISTORY: Adenoma.

SPECIMEN RECEIVED: Cecal ascending polyp.

GROSS DESCRIPTION: Received in a container labeled "cecal ascending polyp" are three fragments of tan tissue measuring 0.3 to 0.4 cm diameter. The specimen is totally submitted.

MICROSCOPIC DESCRIPTION: The cecum and ascending mucosal fragments show glands that vary in size and configuration and are lined by uniform epithelial cells. Hyperplasia of the glandular and surface epithelium are prominent with serrated architectures evident.

DIAGNOSIS: Cecum and ascending colon biopsies, mucosal (three): Hyperplastic polyps (three).

Copyright © 2016 by Elsevier Inc.

57. FROM OPERATIVE REPORT 43

CLINICAL HISTORY: Lumbar herniated disc.

TISSUE RECEIVED: Lumbar disc.

GROSS DESCRIPTIONS: Submitted in formalin, labeled with the patient's name and "lumbar disc" are several irregular fragments of pink-tan ragged tissue measuring approximately 2 × 1.5 × 0.5 cm in aggregate. Submitted in toto.

MICROSCOPIC DESCRIPTIONS: The slide shows several irregular fragments of fibrocartilaginous intervertebral disc material. There are no significant inflammatory infiltrates or evidence of neoplasm.

DIAGNOSIS: Intervertebral disc, lumbar region, discectomy: fragments of intervertebral disc.

58. PATHOLOGY REPORT

SPECIMEN RECEIVED: A. polyps, cecum/sigmoid—adenoma. B. Barrett's esophagus—rule out dysplasia.

GROSS DESCRIPTION: The specimens are received in two containers:

A. In the container labeled "colon biopsy and polyp" are four fragments of tan-pink tissue measuring 0.3 to 0.6 cm diameter. The specimen is totally submitted as "A."
B. In the container labeled "Barrett's esophagus biopsy" are six fragments of tan-gray tissue measuring 0.1 to 0.3 cm diameter. The specimen is totally submitted.

MICROSCOPIC DESCRIPTION:

A. The mucosal fragments of the cecum and sigmoid colon show polypoid architectures with adenomatous features within surface and glandular epithelial sites. The glands vary in size and configuration and are lined by enlarged, mildly pleomorphic cells with elongated hyperchromatic nuclei.
B. The esophageal biopsies demonstrate gastric cardia mucosa exhibiting intestinal metaplasia. The glands vary in size and configuration and have uniform elongated epithelial cells. Separation by a fibrous lamina propria is evident.

DIAGNOSIS:

A. Cecum and sigmoid colon biopsies, mucosal: Adenomatous polyp fragments.
B. Esophageal biopsy: Gastric cardia mucosa with intestinal metaplasia, consistent with Barrett's esophagus.

59. FROM OPERATIVE REPORT 14

SPECIMEN RECEIVED: Muscle biopsy, left deltoid.

INDICATION: Lipoma left posterior axillary fold.

GROSS DESCRIPTION: Received in a container labeled "muscle biopsy left deltoid" is a fragment of brown tissue measuring 0.7 × 0.5 × 0.5 cm. The specimen is totally submitted.

MICROSCOPIC DESCRIPTION: The skeletal muscle of the left deltoid shows normal morphology.

DIAGNOSIS: Muscle biopsy, left deltoid: No pathologic diagnosis.

60. FROM OPERATIVE REPORT 7

CLINICAL HISTORY: Mass of axillary fold.

SPECIMEN RECEIVED: Lipoma from axillary fold.

GROSS DESCRIPTION: The specimen is labeled with the patient's name and "lipoma from axillary fold, intramuscular," which consists of a loosely encapsulated yellow adipose tissue, 8 × 7.8 × 1.8 cm. Sectioning reveals homogeneous yellow adipose tissue throughout. Representative sections in 4 cassettes.

MICROSCOPIC DIAGNOSIS: Mature adipose tissue consistent with lipoma, axillary fold.

61. PATHOLOGY REPORT

CLINICAL DIAGNOSIS AND HISTORY: Cyst.

TISSUE(S) SUBMITTED: Lesion, back.

GROSS DESCRIPTION: Specimen is received in fixative and consists of a 3.3 × 2.5 × 2.2-cm thin-walled cyst containing charcoal, gray-black, friable material.

MICROSCOPIC DESCRIPTION: One microscopic slide examined.

DIAGNOSIS: Follicular cyst, infundibular type, skin of back.

62. FROM OPERATIVE REPORT 12

CLINICAL HISTORY: Left ischial ulcer.

SPECIMEN RECEIVED: Ischial tissue *(left)*.

GROSS DESCRIPTION: Received in a container labeled "left ischial tissue" is an irregularly shaped fragment of soft tissue with a small portion containing an ellipse of skin. The specimen measures 18 × 7.5 × 6 cm in greatest dimension. The skin ellipse measures 4.5 × 2.5 × 0.3 cm. A central opening measuring 2 cm in greatest dimension is present. The remainder of the tissue has a nodular solid tan-gray to brown appearance. On sectioning diffuse fibrosis extends through the area. Representative portions are submitted.

MICROSCOPIC DESCRIPTION: The soft tissue of the left ischial region demonstrates extensive diffuse fibrosis with mild infiltrates of mononuclear inflammatory cells. A significant portion of the soft tissue is covered with granular fibrin containing sheets of neutrophils that rest upon a granulation tissue base. The adjacent epidermis shows pseudoepitheliomatous hyperplasia and normal maturation pattern.

DIAGNOSIS: Skin and soft tissue of left ischial region, excision: Granulation tissue, extensive, with diffuse fibrosis and mild chronic inflammation. Ulcer with mild to moderate acute inflammation.

Copyright © 2016 by Elsevier Inc.

63. FROM OPERATIVE REPORT 39

CLINICAL HISTORY: Morbid obesity.

SPECIMEN RECEIVED: Liver biopsy.

GROSS DESCRIPTION: The specimen is labeled with the patient's name and "liver biopsy" and consists of a 2 cm needle core of greenish tissue.

MICROSCOPIC DESCRIPTION: Sections show liver showing mild fatty change. The portal triads are unremarkable.

DIAGNOSIS: Liver biopsy showing mild fatty change.

64. FROM OPERATIVE REPORT 6

CLINICAL DIAGNOSIS AND HISTORY: Cyst.

TISSUE(S) SUBMITTED: Scalp cyst.

GROSS DESCRIPTION: Specimen is received in fixative and consists of an ovoid, rubbery, gray-white, 2 × 1.3 cm diameter cyst with gray-white laminated, friable contents.

MICROSCOPIC DESCRIPTION: One microscopic slide examined.

DIAGNOSIS: Follicular cyst, isthmus-catagen type (pilar cyst), clinically scalp.

65. FROM OPERATIVE REPORT 19

CLINICAL HISTORY: Left upper lobe abscess—probably secondary aspiration, culture and pseudomonas.

SPECIMEN RECEIVED: Lung, left upper lobe.

GROSS DESCRIPTION: Received in a container labeled "left upper lobe of lung" is a lung upper lobe measuring 17 × 11 × 3.4 cm as a collapsed specimen. The lobe weighs 283 grams. All surfaces have a dull gray yellow exudate that extends over the pleura. The pleura has a wrinkled collapsed appearance. On sectioning the majority of the lung parenchyma is replaced by a necrotic collapsed cyst with a ragged gray-yellow wall. This completely encompasses the vast majority of lung parenchyma with only small portions persisting in the base of the upper lobe. Bronchus and vascular structures are identified and appear unremarkable. Multiple representative sections of lung parenchyma are submitted.

MICROSCOPIC DESCRIPTION: The left upper lobe tissue sections show an extensive area of coagulation necrosis and marked destruction of the pulmonary parenchyma. Sheets of neutrophils are present within fibrin and coagulation necrosis debris. The adjacent lung tissue shows collections of macrophages and inflammatory cells within alveoli. Abundant fibrin debris accompanies the inflammation. Prominent squamous metaplasia is present within the bronchial tree that persists. Extensive interstitial fibrosis within the adjacent lung parenchyma is also present.

DIAGNOSIS: Lung, left upper lobe, resection: Abscess, large, with severe acute inflammation and extensive necrosis. Interstitial fibrosis with chronic inflammation, adjacent lung tissue.

Copyright © 2016 by Elsevier Inc.

66. FROM OPERATIVE REPORT 21

CLINICAL HISTORY: Atelectasis lung.

GROSS DESCRIPTION: 20 ml of mucoid fluid received in one container.

SPECIMEN RECEIVED: Bronchial washing.

SPECIMEN ADEQUACY: Specimen satisfactory for cytologic evaluation.

DIAGNOSIS: Atypical cells, cannot rule out malignancy.

COMMENTS: Rare groups of mildly atypical squamous cells present, significance and origin unknown. Cytology correlated with accompanying histology specimen. Please see pathology report.

Report amended due to transcription error on original. Discussed with Dr. Green.

67. FROM OPERATIVE REPORT 23

CLINICAL HISTORY: Pleural effusion, unknown cause.

GROSS DESCRIPTIONS: Ten ml bloody fluid received in one syringe.

SPECIMEN RECEIVED: Pleural fluid.

SPECIMEN ADEQUACY: Specimen satisfactory for cytologic evaluation.

DIAGNOSIS: No cytologic evidence of malignancy.

COMMENTS: Specimen shows predominantly lymphocytes.

68. 2/1/XX FAMILY PRACTICE SERVICE, MARK ADAMS, MD

(REPORTS 68 TO 79 ARE FOR THE SAME PATIENT)

This 68-year-old female presents to the office today requesting a complete physical examination. She recently moved to our area and states that she would like to establish with a family practitioner. She has a history of coronary artery disease, status post coronary artery bypass × 3 in 1978. She has been doing well. Gravid 3, para 3, postmenopausal about 20 years. History is also significant for hypertension, controlled by diet. Otherwise no complaints.

PAST MEDICAL HISTORY: Remarkable for conditions stated above.

OPERATIONS:

1. Hysterectomy with bladder repair, 1973
2. Bilateral blepharoplasty
3. D&C × 4

ALLERGIES: None.

MEDICATIONS: Digoxin 0.25 mg, Lasix 40 mg p.o. q.d., estrogen.

TOBACCO: Does not smoke.

ALCOHOL: Occasional.

SOCIAL HISTORY: Homemaker, mother of three. Husband recently transferred to area from California.

Copyright © 2016 by Elsevier Inc.

FAMILY HISTORY: Mother deceased from heart disease. Father has had multiple strokes. Two brothers, one with polio. Three children, health good. One sister, died of breast cancer at age 35.

REVIEW OF SYMPTOMS: Denies nausea, vomiting, headaches, dysuria, incontinence, dyspnea. Occasional bouts of atrial fibrillation; always converts spontaneously.

HEENT: Wears glasses. Otherwise negative.

RESPIRATORY: Negative.

CARDIOVASCULAR: Negative except as discussed above.

GI/GU: Postmenopausal, on estrogen.

ENDOCRINE: No diabetes or thyroid problems.

MUSCULOSKELETAL: Some arthritis, both hands.

PSYCHIATRIC: Negative.

PHYSICAL EXAMINATION: Reveals a very pleasant elderly female in no distress.

VITALS: Blood pressure is 140/84 right arm sitting position, 150/90 left arm sitting position; pulse 90 and regular.

WEIGHT: 115 lb.

SKIN: No skin lesions are present.

NODES: No lymphadenopathy.

ENT: Negative.

CHEST: Clear to auscultation.

CARDIAC: Reveals a regular rhythm. I did not hear any murmurs or gallops.

BREAST EXAMINATION: Right side free from lumps or masses. Small lump noted in left breast on examination, which is painless, without discharge, without retraction.

ASSESSMENT AND PLAN:

1. History of coronary artery disease, status post coronary artery bypass. No complaints at present, no abnormal findings. Continue medications as previously prescribed.
2. Breast mass on examination. Suggest mammography. If positive, consultation will be requested from surgery.
3. Postmenopausal, continue on estrogen therapy.

69. 2/2/XX JACOB BOND, MD

Patient has bilateral diagnostic mammography that shows normal finding on the right but dense, suspicious area on the left. Suggestion by radiologist is further clinical study.

Copyright © 2016 by Elsevier Inc.

70. 2/5/XX JACOB BOND, MD

Patient is seen today in the clinic at the request of Dr. Adams for evaluation of suspicious lump in the left breast. Patient states that she does not practice self-breast examination and therefore was unaware of the existing lump. She does state, however, on reflection, that the left breast at times was painful. No nipple discharge or puckering has been noted. Patient states that she has a sister who died of breast cancer in her mid-thirties. No other family history for cancer was noted.

EXAMINATION: Both breasts seem to be symmetrical. No abnormal findings on first view, right breast examination benign. Left breast identifies small lump where calcifications were noted on mammography.

ASSESSMENT: Left breast mass.

PLAN: Although it is difficult to say that this is not a single cyst, I would recommend a breast biopsy at patient's earliest convenience to rule out any possible malignancy. Options to include conservative measures of waiting for further signs, repeat mammography, 6-month breast checks were discussed with patient as well as risks and benefits of biopsy and possible mastectomy if findings are positive. Patient wishes to discuss with her husband and will let me know what she decides.

Thank you for asking me to consult on the care of Mrs. Smith. My recommendations are as above. I will await her further decision if she wishes further care from a surgical standpoint.

71. 2/8/XX JACOB BOND, MD

Phone call from patient wishing to schedule left breast biopsy. Scheduled for 2/10/XX by Dr. Bond.

72. 2/10/XX JACOB BOND, MD (ADMISSION SERVICE)

This patient is a 68-year-old female with chief complaint of left breast mass, admitted for left breast biopsy. The patient has a history of hypertension, coronary artery disease, and coronary artery bypass × 3. She also has a history of hysterectomy and is on estrogen therapy. She was in her usual state of health until a physical examination in early February, which revealed a small mass in the left breast. Mammography reportedly confirmed presence of mass and calcifications. Right breast exhibited no abnormal findings. The patient had menarche at age 12 and has given birth to three children. The patient has a family history positive for one sister with breast carcinoma. Medical history: as stated above for hypertension and CAD.

PHYSICAL EXAMINATION: Reveals a well-developed, well-nourished female in no apparent distress. The vital signs are stable, afebrile. The HEENT examination is within normal limits. The neck is supple, and the trachea is midline. No masses or adenopathy are present. The lungs are clear to auscultation and percussion. The cardiovascular examination is within normal limits. The left breast exhibits the presence of a small mass. The right breast is within normal limits. The right axilla is normal without adenopathy. The left axilla reveals small, less than 1 cm nonfixed, no matted lymph nodes. The abdominal examination is within normal limits. The rectal examination is normal, with guaiac-negative stool present in the vault.

Copyright © 2016 by Elsevier Inc.

ASSESSMENT: Left breast mass, admitted for breast biopsy and possible mastectomy.

73. 2/10/XX JACOB BOND, MD

Excisional breast biopsy was performed using local anesthesia. Pathology report documented adenocarcinoma of left breast. Patient was taken to operating room, administered general anesthesia, and underwent surgery the same day for mastectomy.

74. 2/10/XX JACOB BOND, MD

PREOPERATIVE DIAGNOSIS: Carcinoma of the left breast.

POSTOPERATIVE DIAGNOSIS: Same.

PROCEDURE PERFORMED: Left total mastectomy and left axillary node dissection. *(This is a modified radical mastectomy.)*

HISTORY: Patient underwent left breast biopsy for suspicious lesion 2/10/XX. Pathology report returned with diagnosis of adenocarcinoma of breast. Patient and her family discussed the benefits of the proposed total mastectomy and the risks, including death. Patient gives her understanding and agrees to proceed with the proposed procedure.

PROCEDURE: With the patient in the supine position under good general endotracheal anesthesia, a folded towel was placed beneath her left scapula and her left arm abducted on a pillow. She was prepped thoroughly with Betadine; the extent of her mastectomy incision was marked with a marking pen. We went about half an inch superior and half an inch inferior to her most medial circum-mammary incision, and it was a transverse incision. The draping was completed with Minnesota Mining drape and sterile paper in the usual manner. The superior flap was raised first. Bleeders on the breast were clamped and bovied; small bleeders on the flap were clamped and tied with 3-0 silk. The superior flap was raised to the clavicle inferior to the rectus sheath, medially to the sternal border, and laterally to the latissimus dorsi. The breast was outlined with a bovie, and then the breast was removed medially and laterally. We were somewhat concerned about involving the pectoralis muscle here, but it did not, and we could not see any invasion to the pectoralis fascia. Perforators were clamped and oversewn with 2-0 silk figure-of-eights. Small bleeders on the pectoralis major were bovied. The breast was allowed to fall laterally. The clavipectoral fascia was taken down. There was an area of scar tissue on the superior lateral portion of the pectoralis major attached to the breast, and we thought this was in the area of the previous biopsy. We had to dissect this off sharply, and it did not appear to be a cancer. Then she had a lot of inflammatory tissue in the axilla, which was rather difficult to define, but we exposed the axillary vein, hemoclipped the small venous tributaries, and dissected the axilla down to the 7th rib, and then took the breast off the serratus by bovie; the lateral chest bleeders were clamped and tied with 3-0 silk. The axilla was inspected, and the long thoracic and thoracodorsal nerve was intact. We left the superior branch of the intercostal brachial. It was dry. The mastectomy site was lavaged out with a liter of sterile water. Small bleeders were bovied. Several bleeders on the flaps were clamped and tied with 3-0 silk. The chest tubes were placed in the axilla and over the pectoralis major and exited laterally inferiorly, and the flaps were brought together without any tension

Copyright © 2016 by Elsevier Inc.

with pulley sutures of 2-0 silk; then the wound was closed with a running 4-0 Prolene vertical mattress suture, removing the pulley sutures as we went. Vaseline dressings and dry dressings were applied.

Estimated blood loss was 400 ml. She tolerated this well. The flaps seemed to be intact. The drains were sewn into place and dry dressings applied. She tolerated the procedure well and was returned to the recovery room in good condition.

75. 2/12/XX JOYCE HARKNESS, MD, CONSULTING PHYSICIAN

CHIEF COMPLAINT: Atrial fibrillation.

Patient is a 68-year-old female, status post left total mastectomy for carcinoma of left breast. She has been doing fairly well postoperatively until this morning when she awoke with complaints of fluttering in the chest. ECG shows periods of rapid atrial fibrillation, with conversion to sinus rhythm spontaneously.

Past history is positive for CAD and hypertension. Patient is status post coronary artery bypass × 3. No chest pain or anginal symptoms have been noted.

Cardiac examination at present shows regular rate and rhythm; no gallops or murmurs are noted.

ASSESSMENT: Atrial fibrillation, status post left total mastectomy.

RECOMMENDATION: Treat conservatively with Coumadin at present. Monitor closely for signs of rhythm not converting spontaneously. Consideration would then have to be given to converting medically. Electrocardioversion is not recommended at this time.

76. 2/14/XX ANTHONY CASH, MD, CONSULTING PHYSICIAN

CHIEF COMPLAINT: Second-opinion surgery consultation *(inpatient)* regarding acute onset of no palpable pulses in lower extremities.

Mrs. Smith is a 68-year-old female with known history of CAD, status post coronary bypass in the 1970s. She recently underwent a total mastectomy 2/10/XX by Dr. Bond. Postoperatively, the patient has had an unremarkable course. Diet and activity were gradually increased. This morning she got up from bed about 4:30 and was weighed and had no problems. About 6:30 she suddenly experienced an acute onset of bilateral leg pain. The pain was excruciating. She was lying in bed when this first occurred. The surgical service was consulted about 7:30 this morning. By history from the patient, the pain gradually decreased. At the time of initial examination, she was complaining of a greater pain in her left thigh. She did state that her right leg had more of a numb feeling. She claimed that both legs were heavy feeling and that she would have to move every now and then to get relief from the pain.

Pertinent history reveals that the patient has been intermittently in atrial fibrillation. She has received two doses of Coumadin postoperatively for this atrial fibrillation.

Initial examination of the patient reveals a well-developed, well-nourished white female in no apparent distress. Heart: Regular rate and rhythm. Lungs are clear to auscultation bilaterally. Chest: The patient has a well-healing incision. There are no signs of infection, such as erythema or discharge. Abdomen: Positive bowel sounds, soft, nontender, nondistended. No rigidity on palpation. Examination of the pulses reveals the following: 2/4 in the radial, 2/4 in the carotid. No palpable pulses from the femoral on

Copyright © 2016 by Elsevier Inc.

down. The patient does have dopplerable pulses in the femorals bilaterally. She has dopplerable left posterior tibial and no dopplerable right dorsalis pedis pulse. Neuro: Cranial nerves II–XII grossly intact.

IMPRESSION: Probable saddle embolus to the distal aorta.

PLAN: Patient in need of emergent embolectomy with possible aortofemoral reconstruction. Acute onset of bilateral leg pain and numbness. Embolism most likely from left atrium. Patient has been in and out of atrial fibrillation postoperatively. Discussed the risks, benefits, and complications of the procedure with the patient. The patient understands she will be cared for postoperatively in the surgical intensive care unit.

Thank you for this interesting consultation. We agree with your initial assessment and are happy to participate in the care of this nice lady.

77. 2/14/XX JACOB BOND, MD

PREOPERATIVE DIAGNOSIS: Saddle embolus, distal aorta.

POSTOPERATIVE DIAGNOSIS: Same.

PROCEDURE PERFORMED: Bilateral aortofemoral embolectomy via femoral artery approach, femoral embolectomy.

PROCEDURE: The patient was placed in the supine position and given a general anesthetic. She was prepped from her nipples to her toes. Following this, two bilateral groin incisions were made and dissection was carried down. The common femoral, profunda femoral, and superficial femoral arteries were identified on both sides and controlled with vessel loops. Following this, starting with the right side, a linear arteriotomy was made over the superficial femoral artery and profunda arteries. No. 3 Fogarty catheters were passed distally down the superficial femoral arteries and profunda arteries. No thrombus was recovered. They were then flushed with heparinized saline and controlled with vessel loops. Following this, no. 4 and no. 6 Fogarty catheters were sequentially placed up the common femoral artery toward the iliofemoral area. A lot of thrombus was removed, and good arterial inflow was established in the right leg. Before any arteriotomies had been made, the patient had been given 5000 units of IV heparin that had been given 5 minutes to circulate.

Following this, the arteriotomy on the right was closed with a running 5-0 Prolene suture. Before the arteriotomy was closed, it was back-flushed and fore-flushed. The clamps and vessel loops were all removed, and flow was restored to the right lower extremity. The patient had dopplerable posterior tibial pulses and palpable dorsalis pedis pulses at this point. Following this, a similar incision was made in the left lower extremity, and catheters were placed distally down the profunda and superficial femoral arteries, also flushing them sequentially with heparinized saline. No thrombus was removed from the distal arteries on the left; following this, no. 4 and no. 6 Fogarty catheters were placed sequentially toward the iliofemoral artery and more thrombotic material was removed, restoring good arterial inflow. The arteriotomy on the left was closed in a similar fashion with running 5-0 Prolene. All the clamps were removed. There were palpable dorsalis pedis and dopplerable posterior tibial pulses at this junction of the procedure. Following this, both wounds were irrigated free of clot and debris. They were closed with three layers of interrupted 3-0 Vicryl, and the skin was closed with staples. The patient tolerated the procedure well and went to the recovery room in good condition.

Copyright © 2016 by Elsevier Inc.

78. 2/17/XX ERIC ARNOLD, MD, CONSULTING PHYSICIAN

REASON FOR CONSULTATION: Pleural effusion.

Patient is a 68-year-old female who was initially admitted for a left breast biopsy. Pathology confirmed carcinoma, and patient proceeded to have left total mastectomy. Hospital course has been complicated by atrial fibrillation and saddle embolism, requiring embolectomy. Patient is now 4 days postop embolectomy and has developed persistent pleural effusion. Attempts at medical management have failed, and patient is developing respiratory failure. A pleuracentesis is accomplished, with 500 ml of blood-tinged fluid immediately aspirated. Patient appears to receive immediate relief. Patient will be closely monitored in intensive care unit for additional signs of respiratory failure.

79. 3/10/XX JACOB BOND, MD

Patient in for follow-up appointment, as status post mastectomy on 2/10/XX. Hospital course was complicated by atrial fibrillation and embolism, requiring embolectomy. Patient also developed pleural effusion requiring pleuracentesis. Patient has now been discharged from the hospital for 10 days. Other than some incisional pain, patient seems to be doing well. No major complaints: denies shortness of breath, nausea, loss of appetite, fever, or pain in extremities. Energy levels seem to be returning to normal. Incision sites are examined, with no erythema or infection noted. Sutures are removed. Patient is instructed not to lift, push, or pull objects and to return to activities slowly. Wound care is reviewed. Patient is instructed to follow-up in 2 weeks or sooner if complaints.

80. PULMONARY FUNCTION STUDY

This 49-year-old presents with dyspnea. He has previous cigarette smoking history.

COMPLETE PULMONARY FUNCTION STUDY: Forced vital capacity is 4.87 L, 112% of predicted. FEV1 is 4.02 L, 113% of predicted. FEV1 is 83%. FEF 25% to 75% is normal. There is no significant response to bronchodilators. Flow volume loop shows a well-preserved inspiratory limb.

Total lung capacity by plethysmography is 6.82 L, 111% predicted. RV/TLC ratio and airway resistance are normal. Corrected DLCO was 18.99, 70% of predicted.

IMPRESSION:

1. Normal expiratory flow rates.
2. Normal lung volumes.
3. Mild reduction of DLCO is noted.

The cause of decreased diffusion capacity is unclear in this patient. Possible causes could include heart disease, pulmonary embolism, anemia, obstructive sleep apnea. Clinical correlation is advised for cause of abnormal diffusion. There is no evidence of coexisting obstructive or restrictive pulmonary disease.

Note: The items to be coded listed below:

- Spirometry before and after bronchodilator
- Respiratory flow volume loop
- Functional residual capacity

Copyright © 2016 by Elsevier Inc.

- Carbon monoxide diffusing capacity
- Bronchodilator supply

81. OPERATIVE REPORT

PREOPERATIVE DIAGNOSIS: History of adenocarcinoma of the prostate.

POSTOPERATIVE DIAGNOSIS: History of adenocarcinoma of the prostate.

PROCEDURES PERFORMED:

1. Transrectal ultrasound performance with:
2. Volume study.
3. Needle localization.
4. Needle implantation.
5. Cystoscopy.

ANESTHESIA: General.

ESTIMATED BLOOD LOSS: Minimal.

PROCEDURE: Please see the preoperative note for indications of the procedure, as well as full informed consent. The patient underwent a general anesthetic and was put in the extended dorsal lithotomy position. The table was decanted or in Trendelenburg 5 degrees. He was prepped and draped in the usual fashion, which included a 14-French Foley catheter with 120 ml of sterile saline in his bladder. The testicles and scrotum had been taped back and away. We irrigated the rectum with sterile saline, performing a pseudo-enema. The patient underwent transrectal ultrasound placement. This was connected to the gantry. The placement of ultrasound and the grid work were set up so that the base of the prostate is noted at #1 on the grid work. The anterior most component at approximately 4.5–5, prostate extended from side-to-side from A to F.

Five-mm increment imaging slices were obtained, starting at the base of the prostate, carrying it back for a total of 3 cm to 30. Volume of the prostate is approximately 33 ml.

The outline of the prostate was drawn during the volume study. This information was given to the computer electronically so that a plan could be developed. Once the plan had been completed, the placement of the needles was performed in the usual fashion. The dose was delivered via 125 seeds after placement of the needles.

The total number of needles was 41 for 107 seeds (radioelements) placed with ultrasound guidance. The patient tolerated this well. At the conclusion, the patient was re-prepped and draped with the Foley catheter being removed and a cystoscopic evaluation was performed. There is no evidence of perforation of the urethra, bladder neck, or bladder. Urine within the bladder was clear. No seeds or spacers could be identified. An 18-French Foley catheter was then placed along with Triple antibiotic salve to the perineum and mesh panties. He tolerated the procedure well overall. Estimated blood loss minimal.

82. OPERATIVE REPORT

PREOPERATIVE DIAGNOSIS: History of a nodular mass, mid-prostate with urinary retention.

Copyright © 2016 by Elsevier Inc.

POSTOPERATIVE DIAGNOSIS: History of a nodular mass, mid-prostate with urinary retention; possible macronodular prostate.

PROCEDURE: Cystoscopy, transurethral resection of the prostate, one stage.

ANESTHESIA: Spinal.

ESTIMATED BLOOD LOSS: Approximately 100 ml.

FINDINGS: Benign prostatic hypertrophy type changes.

This is a 76-year-old gentleman who has a history as outlined in the preoperative note. Cystoscopically there is a large, red, macronodular area along the base of the prostate, which has been noted. The patient is having outlet obstructing symptoms. He has some decompensation in his urinary bladder but in discussion with the findings he wishes to go through the transurethral resection of prostate as outlined and discussed.

The patient underwent a spinal anesthetic, was put in the dorsolithotomy position, prepped, and draped in the usual fashion. Cystoscopic evaluation reveals the 1-cm nodule along the base of the prostate. This appears more macronodular but is not really prostatic or is very minimally prostatic. It could represent a deteriorating median lobe.

Resection of the prostate was started at the 12-o'clock position and was carried between 3 and 9 o'clock back to the plane of the verumontanum. The base tissue and the rest of the lateral walls were then resected. This was a pretty small prostate, around 20 ml of tissue. The area was separately resected.

At the conclusion of this procedure, the chips were irrigated out of the bladder. Final hemostasis was achieved. A 22-French three-way Foley catheter was inserted, inflated, and irrigated with slightly tinged irrigant returning. He was taken to the Recovery Room in satisfactory condition.

83. OPERATIVE REPORT

PREOPERATIVE DIAGNOSIS: History of left cryptorchid testicle.

POSTOPERATIVE DIAGNOSIS: Left ectopic testicle.

PROCEDURE PERFORMED: Left groin exploration with orchiopexy.

ANESTHESIA: General.

Please see the preoperative note for indications of the procedure as well as full informed consent. This 14-year-old was recognized on a sports physical as having a nonpalpable testicle. Through his younger years, it had been palpable.

The testicle on physical exam sat in the superficial inguinal canal next to the external ring. With him asleep, we went ahead and evaluated again and, again, the testicular cord was foreshortened, not allowing the testicle to get into the scrotum proper and sat slightly lateral as noted on the preoperative note.

He underwent a general anesthetic as noted previously and was prepped and draped in the usual fashion. A transverse incision was made halfway between the anterosuperior iliac spine and pubic tubercle at the presumed location of the internal ring. The external oblique aponeurosis was opened along the course of its fibers to the external ring. The inguinal canal was opened. The external ilioinguinal nerve was identified and preserved. The testicle could be identified outside the inguinal canal lateral to it in its own small covering. This was opened and the cord, with the testicle, could be freed up. We removed some of the adhesions along the cord, which allowed

Copyright © 2016 by Elsevier Inc.

very satisfactory length to allow it to fit well into the inferior aspect of the left hemiscrotum.

A separate incision was made in the left hemiscrotum. Subdartos pouch was formed using sharp and blunt dissection. The testicle was brought through in a medial tract performed by using blunt dissection with a hemostat. The testicle was brought down into the scrotum and out of the incision with ease. On the inferior pole of the testicle, a small 3-0 chromic was placed in the inferior most portion of the septum. The scrotal wall was then closed over the testicle with interrupted 3-0 chromic. Irrigation of the wound was performed. No active bleeding could be identified. The external oblique aponeurosis was closed utilizing 3-0 silk. Bupivacaine 0.25% without epinephrine was placed approximately 3 ml in the internal ring and 3 ml in the subcut. The subcut was closed with interrupted 3-0 chromic and 4-0 undyed Vicryl for subcuticular incision closure with Steri-Strips. He tolerated the procedure well.

84. TRANSURETHRAL NEEDLE ABLATION (TUNA) THERAPY

The procedure was performed in the usual fashion and multiple segments as noted.

Transrectal ultrasound was performed with the patient in the left lateral position. The ultrasound is performed in order to evaluate the prostate in detail, bladder neck, and seminal vesicles. Ultrasound shows a width of the prostate at 45 mm. The entire calculated volume of the prostate is approximately 40 cc's. Large amount of the bladder neck/median lobe is noted as prominent. No other findings are noted in the prostate.

A prostatic block was then performed. Using an 83, 18-gauge spinal needle, the area between the "angle" of the prostate to seminal vesicle laterally is identified. Needle is placed into position at that point under the rectum. 8 cc's of 2% Xylocaine are used to create the block.

The patient was then brought to the cystoscopic area. Further preparation includes viscous Xylocaine and liquid Xylocaine to the bladder. After a 15-minute wait, we proceeded with the procedure as follows.

The scope was advanced down into the urethra through the sphincter and prostatic urethra and into the bladder. A prominent bladder neck is noted. The length of the prostate is about 28 mm. The obstructing components are definitely the median lobe.

After introduction of the radiofrequency thermotherapy stylet, treatments were performed utilizing a suggested needle-length of 16 mm.

The treatments were performed 1 cm back from the bladder neck laterally. One cm back from that positioning, the next treatment halfway between the original and the verumontanum. This was performed bilaterally. All target temperatures were reached without difficulty. The fifth treatment zone was the median lobe. We retracted the needles to 12 mm to do this. The patient tolerated the procedure well. Foley catheter was placed at the conclusion of the procedure. Usual post procedure protocol to include antibiotics and pain relief medications.

85. OPERATIVE REPORT

PREOPERATIVE DIAGNOSIS: Glaucoma, severe stage, open angle, right eye.

POSTOPERATIVE DIAGNOSIS: Same.

OPERATION PERFORMED: Sequential cyclocryotherapy, right eye.

Copyright © 2016 by Elsevier Inc.

INDICATION: This 74-year-old white female has an out-of-control glaucoma in her right eye. She is pseudophakic and has been allergic to multiple drops and has had one sequential therapy before that worked quite well and then she stopped taking her drops. It is obvious that despite the cyclocryotherapy, she will need to continue on the Pilocarpine.

DESCRIPTION OF PROCEDURE: After the patient was placed on the OR table, she was given a retrobulbar anesthesia of Xylocaine 2% with 0.75% Marcaine and Wydase for a volume of 3.5 cc. After this, she was prepped and draped in the usual sterile fashion for ophthalmic surgery and a wire lid speculum was used to separate the lids of the right eye. 3.5 mm from the limbus was marked out with a marking pen in the superior temporal quadrant and the right inferior nasal quadrant of her eye. The cryoprobe was liquid nitrogen and nitrous oxide and was applied to –80 for a 5-second treatment in a freeze-thaw-freeze triple row of cryotherapy laid down in both the defined quadrants. There were no complications. Maxitrol ointment, Telfa, and two pads were applied and the patient sent to the Recovery Room.

86. OPERATIVE REPORT

PREOPERATIVE DIAGNOSES:

1. Blunt trauma with paint ball, right eye.
2. Hyphema, right eye, secondary to #1.
3. Recurrent hyphema, right eye, secondary to #1.
4. Corneal staining, right eye, secondary to #1.
5. Increased intraocular pressure, right eye, secondary to #l.
6. Dense cataract, right eye, secondary to #1.

POSTOPERATIVE DIAGNOSIS: Same.

PROCEDURE PERFORMED: Irrigation and aspiration of hyphema and blood clot anterior chamber, right eye.

ANESTHESIA: General endotracheal anesthesia.

INDICATION: This 14-year-old white male has had persistent problems since he was hit with a paint ball in his right eye 2 weeks ago. It has not resolved. It has continued to bleed and now it has formed a huge clot. Because of the increase in pain and obvious corneal staining, it was elected to irrigate the clot at this time. No guarantees were made to the mother for vision.

DESCRIPTION OF PROCEDURE: After the patient was prepped and draped in the usual sterile fashion for ophthalmic surgery under general endotracheal anesthesia, a wire lid speculum was used to separate the lids of the right eye. The Super knife was then used in the limbal area to make a 2-mm–wide incision at the 8-o'clock meridian, and the chamber was filled with BSS Plus. Using the Simcoe I&A apparatus, gentle suction, and a push-pull method, the clot was removed and the blood was irrigated. There was no damage done to the lens surface or to the iris and the pupil remained round. Healon was used to help dissolve the clot and make it easier for aspiration. At the end of the procedure, all the Healon and blood clot was removed and the pupil remained round. There was a dense cataract well on its way to hypermaturity already present, but no evidence of any vitreous or subluxation of the lens. The wound was closed with a 10-0 nylon suture, and the knot was buried. Healon was then placed over the cornea because the cornea showed some irregularity secondary to the paint ball explosion. Solu-Medrol was injected inferiorly Sub-Tenon's. Atropine 1% was placed in

Copyright © 2016 by Elsevier Inc.

the eye and Maxitrol ointment and a Telfa pad, patch, and shield applied. The patient was sent to the Recovery Room. There were no complications.

87. OPERATIVE REPORT

PREOPERATIVE DIAGNOSES:

1. Cataract, right eye.
2. Pseudophakia, left eye.
3. Excess myopia, both eyes.
4. Diabetes mellitus.
5. Atrial fibrillation, controlled.
6. Hypothyroidism.
7. Pacemaker for history of bradycardia.

POSTOPERATIVE DIAGNOSIS: Same.

PROCEDURE PERFORMED: Extracapsular cataract extraction, right eye, with insertion of intraocular lens implant, right eye.

ANESTHESIA: MAC anesthesia.

INDICATION: This 86-year-old white female has had progressively decreasing vision in her right eye secondary to a nuclear sclerotic cataract that has reduced her vision to 20/400, which can be corrected to 20/100. She had successful cataract surgery in her left eye a year ago and has returned to 20/40 vision without glasses. She was counseled again as to the type of procedure, the need for medical clearance, anticoagulation regulation, and pacemaker regulation.

PROCEDURE: After the patient was placed on the OR table, she was given Nadbath and Van Lint anesthesia on a 25-gauge needle for a volume of 9 cc of Xylocaine 2% with 0.75% Marcaine and Wydase. The same mixture was administered on a blunt retrobulbar Atkinson needle for a volume of 4 cc without complications. After this, she was prepped and draped in the usual sterile fashion for ophthalmic surgery, and the Honan balloon was placed for four minutes by the clock at 35 mm Mercury. After this, the lid speculum was used to separate the lids of the right eye and a fornix-based flap was raised from 9 o'clock to 3 o'clock and the wet-field cautery was used. There was no excessive bleeding despite the use of the Coumadin. A 69-Beaver blade made a half-thickness O'Malley groove from 9:30 to 2:30 and the Super knife was used to enter the eye at 11 o'clock. The chamber was filled with Healon, and a dry, nonirrigating anterior capsulotomy was performed on a bent 25-gauge needle. The wound was extended with left and right corneal-cutting scissors, and three 8-0 Vicryls were post placed. Using a lens vectis, the nucleus was expressed without capsular rupture or iris prolapse. The post placed sutures were tied down and the Simcoe I&A apparatus was used to clean up excess cortex. It was noted that there was very weak zonular support and positive vitreous pressure. We elected at this point to fill the chamber with Healon, insert a lens glide, and a 14 diopter L122 UV lens was inserted. Miochol was used to bring down the pupil and eight 10-0 nylons were used to close the wound. A peripheral iridectomy was performed at 1 o'clock and there was no evidence of any vitreous. The Healon was left in the eye. The pupil was round and two 8-0 Vicryls closed the conjunctiva. Solu-Medrol was used sub-Tenon's inferiorly, and Pilopine gel, Maxitrol ointment, Telfa, two pads, and an eye shield were applied. There were no complications, and the heart rate was not out of ordinary since it was protected with a magnet.

Copyright © 2016 by Elsevier Inc.

88. OPERATIVE REPORT

PREOPERATIVE DIAGNOSES:

1. History of corneoscleral laceration, right eye.
2. History of retained sutures, right eye.

POSTOPERATIVE DIAGNOSIS: Same.

PROCEDURE PERFORMED: Removal of retained sutures, anterior cornea, right eye.

ANESTHESIA: General anesthesia.

INDICATIONS: This 17-year-old white male who suffered a severe injury to his eye with multiple lacerations of his right cornea has now recovered to the point that his vision is correctable with a contact lens to 20/25; however, there is a large amount of suture material, and it was elected to remove the sutures at this time.

PROCEDURE: After the patient was prepped and draped in the usual sterile fashion for ophthalmic surgery and he was under general anesthesia, the lid speculum was used to separate the lids of the right eye. Healon was placed over the sutures, a Super knife was used to cut them, and they were pulled with a combination of straight tiers and 0.12 forceps. One suture remained deeply buried and was left alone. None of the scleral sutures were removed. There were no complications and the chamber remained intact. He was patched with TobraDex ointment without Telfa for 24 hours, and we will make arrangements to see him within the week.

89. OPERATIVE REPORT

PREOPERATIVE DIAGNOSIS: Splenic hematoma.

POSTOPERATIVE DIAGNOSIS: Same.

PROCEDURE PERFORMED: Splenectomy.

ANESTHESIA: General.

PROCEDURE: A surgical technique was used to remove the spleen due to splenic hematoma following trauma in football game, kicked. The patient was given general anesthesia. The anesthesiologist inserted a temporary tube into the patient's stomach to empty it. This helped to decompress the stomach and prevent postoperative nausea. A catheter was inserted into the bladder to drain the urine. Surgery was done with the patient lying flat on his back. Several small incisions were made into the abdomen. One was used for the laparoscope, which was attached to a camera that sent images to the video monitor. The other incisions were used to hold or manipulate tissue in the abdomen. Carbon dioxide gas is insufflated into the abdominal cavity to allow room to work and to allow visualizing the area. Parts of the spleen were freed from surrounding tissue. Blood vessels to the stomach and spleen were visualized, clipped with metal clips, and divided. Once the spleen was dissected free of its attachments in the abdominal cavity, it was placed in a special surgical plastic bag and removed through one of the small abdominal incisions. At the end of the surgery, carbon dioxide gas was removed. The small incisions were closed with suture, the skin cleaned, and the incisions covered with a small dressing. Patient tolerated the procedure well.

Copyright © 2016 by Elsevier Inc.

90. RECORD OF OPERATION

PREOPERATIVE DIAGNOSIS: Prostate cancer.

POSTOPERATIVE DIAGNOSIS: Same.

PROCEDURE PERFORMED: Cryoablation of prostate including suprapubic catheter insertion, transrectal ultrasound for prostate volume determination, placement of probes, and guidance of tissue ablation. Suprapubic catheter insertion.

CLINICAL NOTE: This gentleman has had prostate cancer. He has elected to proceed with cryoablation.

PROCEDURE NOTE: The patient was given a spinal anesthetic, prepped and draped in the lithotomy position. The Foley catheter placed into the bladder and transrectal ultrasound probe introduced. Prostate measurements and volumes were determined. Using the Cryoguide system, an 8 probe freeze was selected. Probes were placed under ultrasound guidance. Once all temperature monitors and Cryoprobes were placed the Foley catheter was withdrawn and patient then cystoscoped using the flexible instrument. This ensured the needles had not violated the urethra and the probes were in good position. A 12 French suprapubic catheter was then placed using a trocar technique under endoscopic and ultrasound guidance into the anterior wall of the bladder using a single pass technique. Once probe position was confirmed the urethral warming catheter was placed over a guide wire. A two cycle freeze was undertaken, please see the details. Temperature was recorded in the operative part of the chart. Ice bulb was monitored on ultrasound guidance. At the end of the procedure Cryoprobe was withdrawn. A Foley catheter was placed because of hematuria. CBI was started. Five minutes of pressure was applied to the perineum. Bacitracin ointment was applied to the perineum. The patient tolerated the procedure well and was transferred to the recovery room in good condition.

91. CLINIC PROCEDURE

PREOPERATIVE DIAGNOSIS: Left shoulder bursitis

POSTOPERATIVE DIAGNOSIS: Same

PROCEDURE PERFORMED: Left shoulder injection

PROCEDURE: After obtaining consent, the patient was brought to the Special Procedures area. His left shoulder area was cleaned with Betadine. 7 cc of lo lidocaine and 1 cc of Kenalog were injected in his left subacromial bursa without complications. The patient was slightly nauseated. His blood pressure was 168/107. Heart rate was 79/minute and regular.

I was planning on injecting his right shoulder, however, because of his symptoms I elected to withhold that at this time and do it at some other time.

92. REPORT OF OPERATION

PREOPERATIVE DIAGNOSIS: Left renal calculus.

POSTOPERATIVE DIAGNOSIS: Same.

PROCEDURE PERFORMED: Left ESWL *(extracorporeal shock wave lithotripsy).*

Copyright © 2016 by Elsevier Inc.

CLINICAL NOTE: This gentleman came in with renal colic, a stent was placed. He presents now for ESWL. The patient was given a general laryngeal mask anesthetic, prepped and draped in the supine position. Stone targeted and shock head engaged. A total of 2400 shocks at maximum KV and stone partial fragmentation and dissolution could be seen. The patient tolerated the procedure well and transferred to the recovery room in good condition. He will be seen in follow-up in two weeks' time for KUB.

93. REPORT OF OPERATION

PREOPERATIVE DIAGNOSIS: Acute renal failure, possible rejection, possible ischemic nephropathy.

POSTOPERATIVE DIAGNOSIS: Same.

PROCEDURE PERFORMED: Transplant kidney biopsy.

PROCEDURE: The transplant kidney in the right iliac fossa was visualized with ultrasound. The previous arteriovenous malformation was noted in the lower pole. We avoided that area as much as we could. At least three core biopsies were obtained after prepping the area in the usual fashion and injecting 1% Lidocaine. A post biopsy ultrasound showed no evidence of hematoma or new AVN. The patient had some pain after the procedure and was sent to the procedure area. She will be getting some intravenous morphine.

Hemoglobin will be done in six hours.

94. WALKING OXYGEN DESATURATION STUDY

ENTRANCE DIAGNOSIS: Dyspnea. He gave a board rating of 5 by the time he finished; it was 3 at the beginning and showed some discomfort or effort to do this. He was able to walk 6 minutes at a slow pace without stopping. He did have some wheezing, some coughing, and was able to go 300 feet, which for this age group is relatively poor exercise tolerance. The 02 sats never dropped below 92%.

This patient does not need oxygen therapy with this form of exercise.

95. CLINIC PROGRESS NOTE

SUBJECTIVE: This is a 42-year-old Caucasian female who presents to the clinic today to establish with me as her primary care provider. At this particular visit she is complaining of right hip pain. She also complains of a nagging dry cough and would like to find out what might possibly be causing that. Her right hip pain has been going on for about three months now, which is constant and is aggravated by standing up from sitting. She does not feel the pain as much when walking and she says that this pain sometimes radiates to the buttocks and all the way down to her heel area. She occasionally feels a tingling sensation at the lateral aspect of the thigh, particularly at night. She has been treating this with over-the-counter pain medication but that is not found to be helpful. In terms of her cough, she noticed that she usually gets this whenever she has heartburn.

PAST MEDICAL HISTORY is remarkable for:

1. Gastroesophageal reflux disease and has been taking medication for this but she cannot recall the name of that medication right now.

Copyright © 2016 by Elsevier Inc.

2. She also was found to have only one kidney and this was thought to be congenital.
3. Obesity.

PAST SURGICAL HISTORY is remarkable for a hysterectomy due to a bicornuate uterus.

SCREENINGS: She gets a Pap smear and mammogram every year. Last time was last year, which were normal.

ALLERGIES: She otherwise has no known drug allergies.

FAMILY MEDICAL HISTORY: Her father died at the age of 70 from a myocardial infarction. Mother is presently having high blood pressure and is taking medication for her heart. She also has high blood cholesterol. She is presently 67 years old. There is one brother who has spondylitis, and she has a total of three other sisters. One sister has a benign breast tumor.

PERSONAL AND SOCIAL HISTORY: She is married. She has been doing this job for about 11 years now. She denies alcohol use. She has a total of two children. One is 18 years old and one is 6 years old. She had a miscarriage and one stillbirth.

REVIEW OF SYSTEMS: Constitutional: Head and neck, chest and lungs, cardiovascular, gastrointestinal, genitourinary, and extremities are otherwise negative other than what is already mentioned above.

OBJECTIVE FINDINGS: Vital signs: Blood pressure is 110/70. Pulse rate of 88. Weight is 202 pounds. General survey: She is an obese middle-aged lady who is pleasant in no acute distress. Head and neck: Normocephalic and atraumatic. Pink conjunctivae. Pupils are equal, round, and reactive to light and accommodation. Extraocular movements are intact. Neck is supple. No jugular venous distention. No carotid bruit. No thyromegaly. No cervical lymphadenopathy. Chest and lungs: Symmetrical expansion. Clear breath sounds. No roles or wheezes. Cardiovascular: Normal rate and regular rhythm. No murmur and no gallop. Abdomen is obese, soft; normoactive bowel sounds; nontender. No organomegaly. Extremities: She has no edema, cyanosis, or clubbing. Palpable distal pulses. Straight-leg testing on both lower extremities is essentially negative. She has pain on internal rotation of the right hip joint. No pain on external rotation. On the left side internal and external rotation of the hip joints are negative.

ASSESSMENT/PLAN:

1. Hip pain, exact etiology is uncertain but this could be most likely secondary to degenerative joint disease of the hip versus mild trochanteric bursitis. Superficial femoral nerve syndrome is also a consideration but not very likely. Discussed management with Patient and we will just continue to observe for now. I advised her to give us a call when she develops progression of symptoms and referral to Orthopedics might be appropriate if that happens.
2. Cough, dry, probably related to heartburn symptoms.

Copyright © 2016 by Elsevier Inc.

Answers to Odd-Numbered Workbook Questions

CHAPTER 1: REIMBURSEMENT, HIPAA, AND COMPLIANCE

Theory

1. a. persons eligible for disability benefits from Social Security
   b. persons with permanent kidney failure
3. Social Security Administration
5. 80%
7. 12
9. OBRA
11. beneficiaries
13. Medicare Advantage
15. Administrative Simplification
17. National Provider
19. limiting
21. Internet Only
23. Staff
25. Program, All-Inclusive

CHAPTER 2: AN OVERVIEW OF ICD-10-CM

Theory

1. True
3. True
5. False
7. False
9. True

Copyright © 2016 by Elsevier Inc.

Practical

11. d

13. a

15. e

17. a

19. b

21. c

CHAPTER 3: ICD-10-CM OUTPATIENT CODING AND REPORTING GUIDELINES

Theory

1. False

3. False

5. True

7. False

9. False

11. True

13. True

15. False

Practical

17. Congestive heart failure, **I50.9**. The shortness of breath is a symptom of congestive heart failure and is not reported.

19. Hypertension with end stage renal disease, **I12.0**; end stage renal disease, **N18.6**. There is a combination code for hypertension with end stage renal disease. **I12.0** assumes a causal relationship in this scenario. Under code **I12.0** in the Tabular, a notation states "Use additional code to identify the stage of chronic kidney disease (**N18.5, N18.6**)."

21. Acute lower respiratory infection, **J22**. The Excludes2 note indicates both the infection and COPD may be coded, but the infection is the reason for the encounter.

23. Exposure to tuberculosis, **Z20.1**.

25. Abnormal perfusion study, **R94.39**; cardiovascular disease, **I25.10**. The purpose of the visit is the abnormal perfusion study; therefore, it is reported first, followed by the cardiovascular disease.

27. Contusion of the left cheek, **S00.83XA**; fist fight, **Y04.0XXA**. External cause codes are never reported as a first-listed diagnosis.

29. Encounter for insulin pump titration, **Z46.81**

31. Infant, liveborn, twin, born in hospital, **Z38.30**.

33. Abrasion of left upper arm, **S40.812A**.

35. Acute bronchitis, **J20.9**; COPD, **J44.0**; cigarette smoker, **F17.210**.

CHAPTER 4: USING ICD-10-CM

Theory

1. False

3. False

Copyright © 2016 by Elsevier Inc.

5. True
7. True
9. False
11. False
13. False
15. False
17. Heartburn, acid regurgitation, belching, hoarseness in the morning, reflux, pain in chest, trouble swallowing, choking feeling, dry cough
19. Swelling, pain, discoloration, disfiguration
21. Residual: Constrictive Pericarditis
Cause: Tuberculosis infection

Practical

23. **J01.90** (Sinusitis, acute), **J32.9** (Sinusitis [chronic])
25. **J62.8** (Pneumoconiosis, dust, lime)
27. **J14** (Pneumonia, in, Hemophilus influenzae)
29. **I95.9** (Hypotension)
31. **K85.9** (Pancreatitis, acute), **K86.1** (Pancreatitis, chronic)
33. **E83.31, M90.80** (Rickets, vitamin-D-resistant)
35. **K70.11** (Ascites, due to, hepatitis, alcoholic), **F10.288** (Dependence, alcohol, with, specified disorder NEC)

CHAPTER 5: CHAPTER-SPECIFIC GUIDELINES (ICD-10-CM CHAPTERS 1-10)

Theory

1. True
3. True
5. False
7. True
9. True
11. True
13. True
15. True
17. False
19. True

Practical

21. **A41.9** (Sepsis [generalized]), **R65.20** (Sepsis, severe), **N17.9** (Failure, renal, acute), **J96.00** (Failure, respiration, respiratory, acute)
23. **E86.0** (Dehydration), **B19.10** (Hepatitis, B)
25. **J85.2** (Abscess, lung), **B95.62** (Infection, bacterial, as cause of disease classified elsewhere, Staphylococcus, aureus, methicillin resistant [MRSA])
27. **Z09** (Examination, follow-up [routine] [following] surgery), **Q54.9** (Hypospadias). Because this follow-up exam is part of the episode of care in which surgery corrected the hypospadias, the hypospadias is still coded as if it is an active disease. Once all treatment for the surgery is complete, a history of hypospadias would be reported instead.

Copyright © 2016 by Elsevier Inc.

29. **C80.0** (Neoplasm, disseminated, Malignant Primary), **R18.0** (Ascites, malignant)

31. **L03.116** (Cellulitis, lower limb), **E11.65** (Diabetes, type 2, with, hyperglycemia)

33. **O9A.111** (Pregnancy, complicated by, neoplasm, malignant), **C50.912** (Neoplasm, breast, Malignant Primary)

35. **C61** (Neoplasm, prostate, Malignant Primary), **D63.0** (Anemia, in, neoplastic disease)

37. **K56.60** (Obstruction, intestine), **I12.0** (Hypertension, kidney, with stage 5 chronic kidney disease), **N18.5** (Disease, kidney, chronic, hypertensive, stage 5)

39. **C79.31** (Neoplasm, brain NEC, Malignant Secondary), **Z85.3** (History, personal [of], malignant neoplasm, breast), **Z90.12** (Absence, breast(s) [acquired])

41. **D45** (Polycythemia, vera)

43. **T85.614A** (Complication, insulin pump, mechanical, breakdown), **T38.3X1A** (Table of Drugs and Chemicals, Substance, Insulin, Poisoning, Accidental [Unspecified]), **E10.641** (Diabetes, hypoglycemia, with coma)

45. **C34.11** (Neoplasm, lung, upper lobe, Malignant Primary)

47. **I21.3** (Infarct, myocardium [acute], Q wave)

49. **F20.9** (Schizophrenic), **Z91.14** (Noncompliance, with, medication regimen NEC), **F91.8** (Disorder, conduct, specified NEC)

51. **B05.1** (Meningitis, in [due to], measles)

53. **A52.15** (Polyneuropathy, in [due to], syphilis [late]), **A52.77** (Syphilis, joint [late])

55. **G80.2** (Palsy, cerebral, hemiplegic, spastic)

57. **H81.09** (Meniere's disease, syndrome or vertigo)

59. **J81.0** (Edema, lung, acute), **I50.1** (Failure, ventricle, left), **Z99.11** (Dependence, on, ventilator)

Reports

61. **Report 9: C50.111** (Neoplasm, breast, central portion, Malignant Primary)

63. **Report 20: C79.82** (Neoplasm, endocervix, Malignant Secondary), **C80.1** (Neoplasm, unknown site or unspecified, Malignant Primary)

65. **Report 39: E66.01** (Obesity, morbid), **K76.0** (Fatty, liver), **Z68.42** (BMI, adult, 45.0–49.9)

67. **Report 42: H02.41** (Blepharoptosis), **H53.461** (Hemianopia, homonymous)

69. **Report 90: C61** (Neoplasm, prostate [gland], Malignant Primary)

CHAPTER 6: CHAPTER-SPECIFIC GUIDELINES (ICD-10-CM CHAPTERS 11-14)

Theory

1. True
3. True
5. False
7. False
9. True

Copyright © 2016 by Elsevier Inc.

Practical

11. **K03.2** (Erosion, dental [idiopathic] [occupational] [due to diet, drugs, or vomiting])

13. **N83.6** (Hemorrhage, fallopian tube)

15. **N76.4** (Cellulitis, genital organ NEC, female [external])

17. **N47.2** (Paraphimosis [congenital])

19. **N91.1** (Amenorrhea, secondary)

21. **M79.81** (Hematoma, nontraumatic, soft tissue)

23. **K51.412** (Polyp, polypus, colon, inflammatory, with, intestinal obstruction)

25. **L97.112** (Ulcer, lower limb, thigh, right, with, exposed fat layer)

27. **K40.41** (Hernia, inguinal [internal], with, gangrene, recurrent)

29. **N03.1** (Nephritis, nephritic [focal], chronic, with, focal and segmental glomerular lesions)

31. **L05.02** (Sinus, pilonidal [infected] [rectum], with abscess)

33. **M60.162** (Myositis, interstitial, lower leg)

35. **M32.13** (Lupus, erythematosus, systemic, with organ or system involvement, lung)

37. **M00.242** (Arthritis, streptococcal NEC, hand joint), **B95.1** (Streptococcus, group, B, as cause of disease classified elsewhere)

39. **M60.221** (Granuloma, foreign body [in soft tissue], upper arm)

41. **N61** (Abscess, areola [chronic])

Reports

43. **Report 6: L90.5** (Scar)

45. **Report 10: S14.151A** (Injury, spinal [cord], cervical [neck], posterior cord syndrome, C1 level), **S12.000A** (Fracture, neck, cervical vertebra, first), **S12.100A** (Fracture, neck, cervical vertebra, second), **S12.200A** (Fracture, neck, cervical vertebra, third), **S12.300A** (Fracture, neck, cervical vertebra, fourth), **V47.02XA** (External Cause Index, Accident, transport, car occupant, driver, collision [with], stationary object, non-traffic)

47. **Report 12: L89.224** (Ulcer, pressure, hip)

49. **Report 14: M60.812** (Myositis), **Z99.11** (Dependence, on ventilator)

51. **Report 31: K63.5** (Polyp, colon)

53. **Report 33: N49.3** (Disease, Fournier's); **T18.2XXA** (Foreign body, entering through orifice, stomach)

55. **Report 38: R32** (Incontinence), **Z85.46** (History, personal, malignant neoplasm, prostate)

57. **Report 43: M51.16** (Displacement, intervertebral disc, lumbar, with neuritis, radiculitis, sciatica, or other pain)

59. **Report 92: N20.0** (Calculus, kidney)

CHAPTER 7: CHAPTER-SPECIFIC GUIDELINES (ICD-10-CM CHAPTERS 15-21)

Theory

1. True

3. True

Copyright © 2016 by Elsevier Inc.

5. True

7. True

9. False

11. False

13. True

15. True

17. anomaly

19. abnormal

21. third degree

23. 18

25. severity

Practical

27. **S40.812A** (Abrasion, arm [upper])

29. **T78.2XXA** (Shock, anaphylactic)

31. **O00.9** (Pregnancy, ectopic), **O08.0** (Peritonitis, following ectopic or molar pregnancy)

33. **Q55.64** (Concealed penis)

35. **O26.53** (Pregnancy, complicated by, hypotension)

37. **R13.0** (Aphagia)

39. **S93.402A** (Sprain, ankle)

41. **T23.201D** (Burn, hand[s], right, second degree)

43. **R80.1** (Proteinuria, persistent)

45. **S00.33XD** (Contusion, nose)

47. **Q99.2** (Syndrome, fragile X)

49. **O30.203** (Pregnancy, complicated by, multiple gestations, quadruplet), **Z3A.30** (Pregnancy, weeks of gestation, 30 weeks)

51. **G25.1** (Tremor[s], drug induced), **T43.1X1A** (Table of Drugs and Chemicals, Substance, Monoamine oxidase inhibitor NEC, Poisoning Accidental [unintentional]), **G25.1** (Tremor[s], drug induced)

53. **S60.821A** (Blister, wrist)

55. **S42.001G** (Fracture, traumatic, clavicle)

57. **J80** (Distress, respiratory, adult), **R53.83** (Fatigue)

Reports

59. **Report 28: O76** (Delivery, complicated, by, fetal, heart rate or rhythm), **O66.0** (Delivery, complicated, by, obstruction, due to, dystocia, shoulder), **O70.1** (Delivery, complicated, by, laceration, perineum, second degree), **Z3A.38** (Pregnancy, weeks of gestation, 38 weeks), **Z37.0** (Outcome of delivery, single liveborn).

61. **Report 40: T15.01XA** (Foreign body, cornea)

63. **Report 95: M25.551** (Pain[s], joint, hip), **R05** (Cough)

CHAPTER 8: INTRODUCTION TO CPT

Theory

1–4. any of the following: service or procedure, anatomic site, condition or disease, synonym, eponym, abbreviation

5. d

Copyright © 2016 by Elsevier Inc.

7. b
9. Radiology
11. American Medical Association, or AMA
13. stand-alone code
15. CPT codes and/or HCPCS codes
17. 1966
19. Health Insurance Portability and Accountability Act, or HIPAA

Practical

Radiology

21. 77799
23. 77499

Pathology and Laboratory

25. 81099

Medicine

27. 96999

CHAPTER 9: INTRODUCTION TO THE LEVEL II NATIONAL CODES (HCPCS)

Theory

1. Any of the following: procedures, supplies, products, services
3. Any of the following: procedures, supplies, products, services
5. CMS
7. Professional
9. G
11. Q
13. EY
15. Q
17. d
19. e
21. b

Practical

23. J0129
25. A4680
27. V5264
29. E0999
31. G0009

CHAPTER 10: MODIFIERS

Theory

1. A
3. preoperative services/management or preop
5. no

Copyright © 2016 by Elsevier Inc.

Practical

7. -50

ICD-10-CM: **M71.21** (Cyst, Baker's), **M71.22** (Cyst, Baker's)

ICD-9-CM: **727.51** (Cyst, Baker's)

9. -53

ICD-10-CM: **M17.9** (Osteoarthritis, knee), **I95.81** (Hypotension, postoperative)

ICD-9-CM: **715.96** (Osteoarthritis, lower leg), **458.29** (Hypotension, postoperative)

11. -32

ICD-10-CM: **K50.10** (Enteritis, regional, large intestine)

ICD-9-CM: **555.1** (Enteritis, regional, intestine, large)

13. -32

ICD-10-CM: **Z02.6** (Examination, medical, insurance purpose)

ICD-9-CM: **V70.3** (Examination, medical, insurance certification)

15. -76

17. -99

19. -55

21. -FA

CHAPTER 11: EVALUATION AND MANAGEMENT (E/M) SERVICES

Theory

1. c

3. a

5. e

7. b

9. high

11. low

13. elements

15. moderate severity

17. self-limited/minor severity

19. contributory

21. medical record

23. subjective

25. consultation, attending

27. concurrent

29. review of systems

Practical

Office or Other Outpatient Services and Hospital Inpatient Services

31. a. minimal, minimal/none

   b. minimal

   c. straightforward

   d. **99201**

Copyright © 2016 by Elsevier Inc.

33. **99219** (Evaluation and Management, Hospital Services, Observation Care)

35. **99223** (Hospital Services, Inpatient Services, Initial Hospital Care)

    ICD-10-CM: **I21.19** (Infarction, myocardium [acute], ST elevation [STEMI], inferior), **I25.10** (Arteriosclerosis, coronary [artery]), **Z95.5** (Status, angioplasty, coronary artery, with implant)

    ICD-9-CM: **410.41** (Infarct, myocardial, inferior wall), **414.01** (Arteriosclerosis, coronary [artery]), **V45.82** (Status, percutaneous transluminal angioplasty), with implant

37. **99231** (Hospital Services, Inpatient Services, Subsequent Hospital Care)

    ICD-10-CM: **J15.9** (Pneumonia, bacterial)

    ICD-9-CM: **482.9** (Pneumonia, bacterial)

Consultation Services

39. **99243** (Consultation, Office and/or Other Outpatient)

    ICD-10-CM: **R10.2** (Pain, pelvic [female]), **N94.1** (Dyspareunia [female])

    ICD-9-CM: **625.9** (Pain, pelvic [female], **625.0** (dyspareunia [female])

    Note: All three key components must be met for the service to qualify for the higher level code. In this case, only the MDM complexity was of a higher level, requiring the choice of the lower level code.

41. **99253** (New Patient, Inpatient Consultations)

43. **99232** (Hospital Inpatient Services, Subsequent Hospital Care)

    ICD-10-CM: **R21** (Rash)

    ICD-9-CM: **782.1** (Rash)

    Note that adverse effect from a drug would not be reported as the physician is looking for another cause.

45. **99231** (Hospital Inpatient Services, Subsequent Hospital Care)

    ICD-10-CM: **G44.209** (Headache, tension)

    ICD-9-CM: **307.81** (Headache, tension)

47. **99241** (Consultation, Office and/or Other Outpatient, New or Established Patient)

    ICD-10-CM: **K41.91** (Hernia, femoral, recurrent)

    ICD-9-CM: **553.01** (Hernia, femoral, unilateral, recurrent)

49. **99245** (Consultation, Office and/or Other Outpatient, New or Established Patient)

    ICD-10-CM: **M51.06** (Disorder, disc, with myelopathy, lumbar region)

    ICD-9-CM: **722.73** (Myelopathy, due to or with, intervertebral disc disorder, lumbar, lumbosacral)

Emergency Department Services, Nursing Facility, Domiciliary, and Home Services

51. **99282** (Established Patient, Emergency Department Services)

    ICD-10-CM: **S52.539A** (Colles, fracture), **W21.89XA** (External Cause Index, Striking against, other sports equipment), **Y93.64** (External Cause Index, Activity, baseball)

    ICD-9-CM: **813.41** (Colles' fracture [closed]), **E917.0** (Index to External Causes, Striking against or struck accidentally by others, in sports without subsequent fall), **E007.3** (Index to External Causes, Activity, involving other sports, baseball/softball)

Copyright © 2016 by Elsevier Inc.

53. **99342** (Home Services, New Patient)

    ICD-10-CM: **R60.0** (Edema, legs)

    ICD-9-CM: **782.3** (Edema, legs)

    Note that the leg pain is not reported because the medical documentation indicated that the pain was due to the edema.

55. **99309** (Nursing Facility Services, Subsequent Care)

    ICD-10-CM: **R41.0** (Confusion), **R42** (Dizziness), **I69.30** (Sequelae, infarction, cerebral)

    ICD-9-CM: **298.9** (Confusion), **780.4** (Dizziness), **438.9** (Late effect(s), cerebrovascular disease)

57. **99324** (Domiciliary Services, New Patient)

Prolonged Services and Preventive Medicine Services

59. **99205** for the office visit (Office and/or Other Outpatient Services, New Patient) and **99354** and **99355** for Prolonged Services (Prolonged Services)

Services from Throughout the E/M Section

61. **99205** (Office and/or Other Outpatient Services, Office Visit, New Patient)

63. **99234** (Discharge Services, Observation Care)

    ICD-10-CM: **T39.95XA** (Table of Drugs and Chemicals, Analgesic, Adverse Effect), **L29.8** (Pruritus, specified NEC), **R06.02** (Short, breath)

    ICD-9-CM: **698.9** (Pruritus), **786.05** (Short, breath), **E935.9** (Table of Drugs and Chemicals, Analgesics, External Cause, Therapeutic)

65. **99251** (Consultation, Inpatient)

67. **99291** (Critical Care Services, Evaluation and Management), **99292 × 3** (Critical Care Services, Evaluation and Management)

    ICD-10-CM: **J96.90** (Failure, respiratory), **I50.9** (Failure, heart), **J44.1** (Disease, pulmonary chronic obstructive, exacerbation, [acute]), **Z99.11** (Dependence, on, ventilator)

    ICD-9-CM: **518.81** (Respiratory, failure, acute), **428.0** (Failure, heart), **491.21** (Disease, pulmonary, with, exacerbation NEC [acute]), **V46.11** (Status, ventilator)

Reports

69. Report 1: **99283** (Evaluation and Management, Emergency Department)

    ICD-10-CM: **O23.43** (Infection, urinary, complicating pregnancy), **N39.0** (Infection, urinary [tract]), **R60.0** (Edema, legs)

    ICD-9-CM: **646.63** (Infection, urinary, complicating pregnancy), **599.0** (Infection, urinary [tract]), **782.3** (Edema, legs)

71. Report 3: **99212** (Evaluation and Management, Office and Other Outpatient)

    ICD-10-CM: **S93.401A** (Sprain, ankle)

    ICD-9-CM: **845.00** (Sprain, ankle)

73. Report 5: **99232** (Evaluation and Management, Hospital)

Copyright © 2016 by Elsevier Inc.

CHAPTER 12: ANESTHESIA

Theory

1. moderate sedation or conscious sedation
3. base unit
5. preoperative services
7. conversion

Practical

9. P4 (A patient with severe systemic disease that is a constant threat to life)
11. P3 (A patient with severe systemic disease)
13. P2 (A patient with mild systemic disease)
15. **01382** (Anesthesia, Knee)
17. **00144** (Anesthesia, Corneal Transplant)
19. **00124** (Anesthesia, Otoscopy)
21. **01920-P2** (Anesthesia, Cardiac Catheterization)
23. ICD-10-CM: **K57.33** (Diverticulitis, intestine, large, with, bleeding)
    ICD-9-CM: **562.13** (Diverticulitis, with hemorrhage)
25. ICD-10-CM: **E05.00** (Hyperthyroidism, with goiter)
    ICD-9-CM: **242.01** (Goiter, toxic)

Reports

27. Report 7: **00400** (Anesthesia, Arm, Upper)
29. Report 44: **00140** (Anesthesia, Eye)

CHAPTER 13: SURGERY GUIDELINES AND GENERAL SURGERY

Theory

1. Female Genital
3. categories
5. unlisted
7. major
9. yes
11. local
13. general
15. 99070
17. same
19. dehiscence

Practical

21. 10021-69990
23. Operating
25. 42400
27. therapeutic
29. 40799

CHAPTER 14: INTEGUMENTARY SYSTEM

Theory

Integumentary System Terminology

1. b
3. i
5. a
7. f
9. c
11. a
13. i
15. c
17. e
19. f
21. d

Practical

23. **12032** (Repair, Wound, Intermediate), **99070** (Special Services, Supply of Materials)

    ICD-10-CM: **S41.101A** (Wound, open, arm, [upper])

    ICD-9-CM: **884.0** (Wound, open, arm)

    Note: You do not report an E/M code because this is an established patient and the treatment constitutes the main service provided to the patient.

25. **19081-LT** (Breast, Biopsy, with Localization Device, Placement, stereotactic guidance), **99070** (Special Services, Supply of Materials)

    ICD-10-CM: **D48.62** (Neoplasm, breast, Uncertain Behavior)

    ICD-9-CM: **238.3** (Neoplasm, breast, Uncertain Behavior)

    Note: You do not report an E/M code because this is an established patient and the treatment constitutes the main service provided to the patient.

27. **11451** (Hidradenitis, Excision)

    ICD-10-CM: **L73.2** (Hidradenitis)

    ICD-9-CM: **705.83** (Hidradenitis)

29. **11971** (Removal, Tissue Expanders, Skin)

31. **11976** (Removal, Implant, Contraceptive Capsules)

    ICD-10-CM: **Z30.49** (Contraception, device, maintenance, subdermal implantable)

    ICD-9-CM: **V25.43** (Removal, subdermal implantable, contraceptive)

33. **11444** (Excision, Skin, Lesion, Benign) for 4 cm face lesion, **11423-51** (Excision, Skin, Lesion, Benign) for 3 cm neck lesion

    ICD-10-CM: **D23.30** (Neoplasm, skin, face, benign), **D23.4** (Neoplasm, skin, neck, Benign)

    ICD-9-CM: **216.3** (Neoplasm, skin, face, Benign), **216.4** (Neoplasm, skin, neck, Benign)

Copyright © 2016 by Elsevier Inc.

35. **17000** (Destruction, Lesion, Facial), **17003 ¥ 2** (Destruction, Lesion, Facial)

    ICD-10-CM: **L57.0** (Keratosis, actinic)

    ICD-9-CM: **702.0** (Keratosis, actinic)

37. **12035** (Wound, Repair, Legs, Intermediate); **11042-51** (Debridement, Subcutaneous Tissue)

    ICD-10-CM: **S81.801A** (Wound, open, leg), **W09.1XXA** (External Cause Index, Fall, from, off, playground equipment, swing), **W27.1XXA** (External Cause Index, Contact with, garden fork), **Y92.830** (External Cause Index, Place of occurrence, park [public])

    ICD-9-CM: **891.0** (Wound, open, leg), **E884.0** (Index to External Causes, Fall, from, off, playground equipment), **E920.4** (Index to External Causes, Contact with, garden, fork), **E004.9** (Index to External Causes, Climbing), **E849.4** (Index to External Causes, Accident, occurring, park)

39. **17110** (Destruction, Warts, Flat)

    ICD-10-CM: **B07.8** (Wart, Flat)

    ICD-9-CM: **078.19** (Wart)

41. **11000**, **11001** (Debridement, Skin, Eczematous)

    ICD-10-CM: **L30.9** (Eczema)

    ICD-9-CM: **692.9** (Eczema)

43. **16000** (Burns, Initial Treatment)

    ICD-10-CM: **T23.169A** (Burn, dorsum of hand, first degree), **T31.0** (Burn, extent, less than 10 percent), **X16.XXXA** (External Cause Index, Burning, steam, pipe), **Y92.009** (External Cause Index, Place of occurrence, residence)

    ICD-9-CM: **944.16** (Burn, hand, back, first degree), **948.00** (Burn, extent, less than 10 percent); **E924.8** (Index to External Causes, Burning, steam, pipe), **E849.0** (Index to External Causes, Accident, occurring, home, private)

45. **19020** (Mastotomy, Drainage of Abscess)

    ICD-10-CM: **N61** (Abscess, breast)

    ICD-9-CM: **611.0** (Abscess, breast)

Reports

47. Report 7: **21931** (Excision, Tumor, Back/Flank, 3 cm or greater)

    ICD-10-CM: **D17.1** (Lipoma, site, trunk, [skin])

    ICD-9-CM: **214.8** (Lipoma)

    Note: 11406 would not be correct because the report indicates "dissected free of the muscle."

49. Report 9: **19120-RT** (Excision, Breast, Lesion)

    ICD-10-CM: **C50.111** (Neoplasm, breast, central portion, Malignant Primary)

    ICD-9-CM: **174.1** (Neoplasm, breast, central portion, Malignant, Primary)

Copyright © 2016 by Elsevier Inc.

51. Report 12: **15940** (Ulcer, Pressure)

    ICD-10-CM: **L89.224** (Ulcer, pressure, hip)

    ICD-9-CM: **707.04** (Ulcer, pressure, hip), **707.24** (Ulcer, pressure, stage, 4)

    Note: Modifier -22 may be added to 15940 due to the extensive size of the ulcer.

CHAPTER 15: MUSCULOSKELETAL SYSTEM

Theory

Musculoskeletal Terminology

1. d
3. j
5. b
7. c
9. h
11. g

Answer the Following

13. aspiration of a joint
15. fascia lata graft
17. arthroscopy
19. No, the removal is part of the cast service
21. The primary difference is extent. The codes in the musculoskeletal system subsection are of biopsies of deep subcutaneous tissue, muscle and/or bone, whereas the codes in the integumentary system subsection are for skin and subcutaneous tissue.

Practical

23. **29075** (Cast, Elbow to Finger)

    ICD-10-CM: **Z46.89** (Admission, for, orthopedic [cast]), **S52.119D** (Fracture, forearm)

    ICD-9-CM: **V53.7** (Admission [Encounter], for, fitting of, orthopedic [cast]), **V54.12** (Aftercare, fracture, traumatic, arm, lower)

25. **28406** (Fracture, Calcaneus, with Manipulation)

    ICD-10-CM: **S92.009A** (Fracture, tarsal, calcaneus)

    ICD-9-CM: **825.0** (Fracture, calcaneus [closed])

27. **26700** (Metacarpophalangeal Joint, Dislocation, Closed Treatment)

    ICD-10-CM: **S63.269A** (Dislocation, finger)

    ICD-9-CM: **834.01** (Dislocation, finger, metacarpal, distal end)

29. **27520** (Fracture, Patella, Closed Treatment, without Manipulation)

    ICD-10-CM: **S82.009A** (Fracture, patella)

    ICD-9-CM: **822.0** (Fracture, knee cap, closed)

31. **27570** (Manipulation, Knee)

    ICD-10-CM: **S83.116A** (Dislocation, knee, proximal tibia, anterior)

    ICD-9-CM: **836.51** (Dislocation, tibia, proximal, anterior, closed)

33. **21343** (Sinuses, Frontal, Fracture, Open Treatment)

35. **20615** (Aspiration, Cyst, Bone)

Copyright © 2016 by Elsevier Inc.

37. **20822** (Replantation, Digit)
39. **20526** (Injection, Carpal Tunnel, Therapeutic)
    ICD-10-CM: **G56.00** (Syndrome, carpal tunnel)
    ICD-9-CM: **354.0** (Carpal tunnel syndrome)
41. **20665** (Removal, Halo)
43. **21450** (Fracture, Mandible, Closed Treatment, without Manipulation)
45. **29750** (Cast, Wedging)
47. **29520** (Strapping, Hip)
49. **29200** (Strapping, Thorax)
51. **29049** (Cast, Ambulatory, Figure-of-eight, Shoulder)
53. **29860** (Arthroscopy, Diagnostic, Hip)
55. **29877** (Arthroscopy, Surgical, Knee)
57. **29848** (Ligament, Release, Transverse Carpal)
59. **21032** (Excision, Maxillary, Torus Palatinus)

Reports

61. Report 13: **20610-LT** (Injection, Joint)
    ICD-10-CM: **M75.102** (Syndrome, rotator cuff, shoulder)
    ICD-9-CM: **726.10** (Syndrome, rotator cuff, shoulder)
63. Report 15: **25606-LT** (Fracture, Radius, Distal)
    ICD-10-CM: **S52.572A** (Fracture, radius, lower end, intraarticular), **W10.9XXA** (External Cause Index, Fall, from, unspecified, stairs and steps, initial encounter)
    ICD-9-CM: **813.42** (Fracture, radius, lower end, intra-articular), **E880.9** (Fall, from, off, stairs, steps)
65. Report 17: **27244** or **27244-RT** (Fracture, Femur, Subtrochanteric, Plate/Screw Implant)
    ICD-10-CM: **S72.21XA** (Fracture, femur, upper end, subtrochanteric)
    ICD-9-CM: **820.22** (Fracture, femur [closed], subtrochanteric)

CHAPTER 16: RESPIRATORY SYSTEM

Theory

Respiratory Terminology

1. d
3. k
5. b
7. c
9. f
11. m
13. a
15. e

Answer the Following

17. nasal button
19. septoplasty

Copyright © 2016 by Elsevier Inc.

21. posterior
23. transtracheal and cricothyroid
25. 50

Practical

27. **31267** (Antrostomy, Sinus, Maxillary)
29. **31628-RT** (Bronchoscopy, Biopsy), **31632-RT** (Bronchoscopy, Biopsy). Note: Code 31628 is for a single lobe and two lobes were biopsied. Code 31632 is an add-on code reporting the biopsy of the additional lobe.
31. **31575** (Laryngoscopy, Fiberoptic)
33. **30801** (Ablation, Turbinate Mucosa). Note: Code specified unilateral or bilateral.
35. **30115** and **30115-50** (Excision, Nose, Polyp)
37. **31536** (Laryngoscopy, Direct)
39. **31400** (Arytenoidectomy)
41. **31720** (Aspiration, Trachea, Nasotracheal)
43. **31830** (Revision, Tracheostomy, Scar)
45. **32658** (Thoracoscopy, Surgical, with Wedge Resection of Lung)
47. **32800** (Hernia Repair, Lung)
49. **30930** (Fracture, Nasal Turbinate, Therapeutic)
51. **31613** (Tracheostoma, Revision)

    ICD-10-CM: **J95.02** (Tracheostomy, complication, infection), **L03.221** (Cellulitis, neck)

    ICD-9-CM: **519.01** (Tracheostomy [complication], infection), **682.1** (Cellulitis of neck)
53. **32440** (Pneumonectomy)

    ICD-10-CM: **J61** (Asbestosis [occupational])

    ICD-9-CM: **501** (Asbestosis [occupational])
55. **32900** (Ribs, Resection)

    ICD-10-CM: **Q76.6** (Deformity, rib, congenital)

    ICD-9-CM: **756.3** (Deformity, rib, congenital)
57. **32560** (Pleurodesis, Instillation of Agent)

    ICD-10-CM: **C56.9** (Neoplasm, ovary, Malignant Primary), **J91.0** (Effusion, pleura, malignant)

    ICD-9-CM: **183.0** (Neoplasm, ovary, Malignant Primary), **511.81** (Effusion, pleura, malignant)

Reports

59. Report 19: **32480-LT** (Lobectomy, Lung)

    ICD-10-CM: **J85.2** (Abscess, lung)

    ICD-9-CM: **513.0** (Abscess, lung)
61. Report 23: **32554** (Thoracentesis)

    ICD-10-CM: **J90** (Effusion, pleura)

    ICD-9-CM: **511.9** (Effusion, pleural)

Copyright © 2016 by Elsevier Inc.

CHAPTER 17: CARDIOVASCULAR SYSTEM

Theory

Cardiovascular Terminology

1. e
3. b
5. d
7. a
9. i
11. f
13. j
15. d
17. i
19. h
21. n
23. b
25. l

Answer the Following

27. internally or externally, or intracardiac or external
29. epicardial and transvenous
31. no, suture removal is bundled into the pacemaker procedure
33. 24
35. patient-activated event recorder
37. reversible
39. embolus

Practical

41. **33403** (Valvuloplasty, Aortic Valve)
43. **33464** (Tricuspid Valve, Repair)
45. **93000** (Electrocardiography, Evaluation)
47. **92920** (Angioplasty, Coronary Artery, Percutaneous Transluminal)
49. **93010** (Electrocardiography, Evaluation)
51. **37609** (Ligation, Artery, Temporal)
53. **35452** (Angioplasty, Aorta, Intraoperative)
55. **33513** (Bypass Graft, Venous, Coronary)
    ICD-10-CM: **I24.8** (Insufficiency, coronary)
    ICD-9-CM: **411.89** (Disease, heart, ischemic acute, without myocardial infarction)
57. **33967** (Balloon Assisted Device, Aorta)
    ICD-10-CM: **I21.3** (Infarction, myocardium, myocardial [acute]), **R57.0** (Shock, cardiogenic)
    ICD-9-CM: **410.91** (Infarction myocardium myocardial), **785.51** (Shock, cardiogenic)

Copyright © 2016 by Elsevier Inc.

59. **33641** (Repair, Heart, Septal Defect, Atrium)
ICD-10-CM: **Q21.1** (Defect, septal, atrial)
ICD-9-CM: **745.5** (Defect, atrial septal, congenital)

61. **33533** (Bypass Graft, Arterial, Coronary), **33517** (Coronary Artery Bypass Graft, Arterial-Venous), **33530** (Reoperation, Coronary Artery Bypass, Valve Procedure)
ICD-10-CM: **I25.10** (Arteriosclerosis, coronary, artery)
ICD-9-CM: **414.01** (Arteriosclerosis, coronary, artery, native artery)

Reports

63. Report 26: **33533** (Coronary Artery Bypass Graft [CABG], Arterial Bypass)
ICD-10-CM: **I25.10** (Arteriosclerosis, coronary, artery), **I51.9** (Dysfunction, ventricular)
ICD-9-CM: **414.01** (Arteriosclerosis, coronary, artery, native artery), **429.9** (Dysfunction, ventricular)

CHAPTER 18: HEMIC, LYMPHATIC, MEDIASTINUM, AND DIAPHRAGM

Theory

Hemic and Lymphatic Terminology

1. k
3. e
5. g
7. d
9. i
11. c
13. f
15. b
17. h
19. c

Mediastinum and Diaphragm Terminology

21. m
23. j
25. d
27. l
29. k
31. g
33. b

Practical

35. **38720** (Lymphadenectomy, Radical, Cervical)
ICD-10-CM: **C77.0** (Neoplasm, lymph, gland, cervical, Malignant, Secondary), **C50.012** (Neoplasm, breast, nipple, Malignant Primary)
ICD-9-CM: **196.0** (Neoplasm, lymph, gland, cervical, Malignant, Secondary); **174.0** (Neoplasm, breast, nipple, Malignant, Primary)

Copyright © 2016 by Elsevier Inc.

Note: The lymph gland neoplasm is first-listed because it was the reason for the procedure.

37. **38241** (Bone Marrow, T-Cell Transplantation)

ICD-10-CM: **C92.00** (Leukemia, myelogenous)

ICD-9-CM: **205.00** (Leukemia, myelogenous). Fifth digit "0" is added to indicate the leukemia is not in remission.

39. **38230** (Harvesting, Bone Marrow, Allogeneic)

ICD-10-CM: **Z52.3** (Donor, bone, marrow)

ICD-9-CM: **V59.3** (Donor, bone, marrow)

41. **39200** (Resection, Cyst, Mediastinal)

43. **38209** (Transplantation, Stem Cells, Washing)

45. **78195-26** (Nuclear Medicine, Lymph Nodes), **38792-59** (Lymphadenectomy, Injection, Sentinel Node), **38530** (Excision, Lymph Nodes)

CHAPTER 19: DIGESTIVE SYSTEM

Theory

Digestive Terminology

1. b
3. f
5. g
7. a
9. i
11. i
13. e
15. h
17. a

Practical

19. **43194** (Endoscopy, Esophagus, Removal, Foreign Body)
21. **43401** (Esophagus, Repair, Varices)
23. **44345** (Colostomy, External Fistulization, Revision)
25. **42104** (Excision, Lesion, Palate)
27. **42831** (Adenoids, Excision)
29. **49521** (Repair, Hernia, Inguinal)
31. **40650** (Repair, Lip)
33. **42507** (Parotid Duct, Diversion)
35. **43605** (Biopsy, Stomach)
37. **44604** (Suture, Intestines, Large, Wound)
39. **49320** (Laparoscopy, Abdominal, Diagnostic)
41. **99284-25** (Evaluation and Management, Emergency Department), **43752** (Tube Placement, Nasogastric Tube)

ICD-10-CM: **K92.0** (Hematemesis), **R18.8** (Ascites [abdominal]), **D62** (Anemia, due to, blood loss, acute)

ICD-9-CM: **578.0** (Hematemesis), **789.59** (Ascites), **285.1** (Anemia, due to, blood loss, acute)

Reports

43. Report 31: **45384** (Colonoscopy, Removal, Proximal to Splenic Flexure, with Removal, Polyp)

    ICD-10-CM: **K63.5** (Polyp, colon)

    ICD-9-CM: **211.3** (Neoplasm, intestine, colon, Benign)

    Note: The entry listed under "Neoplasm, intestine, cecum, Benign" indicates **K63.5**, the same code as for the benign polyp of the colon and the code is only reported once.

45. Report 33: **44143** (Hartmann Procedure, Open), **43500-51** (Gastrotomy, Foreign Body Removal), **43830** (Gastrostomy, temporary)

    ICD-10-CM: **N49.3** (Disease, Fournier's); **T18.2XXA** (Foreign body, entering through orifice, stomach)

    ICD-9-CM: **608.83** (Fournier's disease, idiopathic gangrene), **935.2** (Foreign body, entering through, orifice, stomach)

47. Report 35: **43752** (Orogastric Tube Placement)

    ICD-10-CM: **K31.84** (Gastroparesis)

    ICD-9-CM: **536.3** (Gastroparesis)

CHAPTER 20: URINARY AND MALE GENITAL SYSTEMS

Theory

Urinary System Terminology

1. d
3. g
5. f
7. k
9. c
11. l
13. i
15. a
17. d
19. f
21. b
23. h

Male Genital Terminology

25. c
27. e
29. b
31. d
33. e
35. f
37. i
39. c
41. c
43. a
45. f

Copyright © 2016 by Elsevier Inc.

47. a

49. d

51. e

53. a

55. d

57. c

Practical

59. **50390** (Aspiration, Cyst, Kidney)

    ICD-10-CM: **N28.1** (Cyst, kidney, solitary, acquired)

    ICD-9-CM: **593.2** (Cyst, kidney, solitary)

61. **52450** (Incision, Prostate, Transurethral)

    ICD-10-CM: **N41.1** (Prostatitis, hypertrophic)

    ICD-9-CM: **600.00** (Prostatitis, hypertrophic)

63. **54650-50** (Orchiopexy, Abdominal Approach)

    ICD-10-CM: **Q53.21** (Nondescent, testicles, bilateral, abdominal)

    ICD-9-CM: **752.51** (Undescended, testis)

65. **50520** (Fistula, Closure, Kidney)

67. **53215** (Urethrectomy, Total, Male)

69. **53270** (Skene's Gland, Excision)

71. **55400** (Vasovasorrhaphy)

73. **54600** (Repair, Testis, Torsion)

75. **54056** (Destruction, Lesion, Penis, Cryosurgery)

77. **55100** (Abscess, Scrotum, Incision and Drainage)

Reports

79. Report 36: **52332-50** or **52332-RT** and **52332-LT** (Cystourethroscopy, Insertion, Indwelling Ureteral Stent)

81. Report 38: **53445** (Insertion, Prosthesis, Urethral Sphincter)

    ICD-10-CM: **R32** (Incontinence), **Z85.46** (History, personal, malignant neoplasm, prostate)

    ICD-9-CM: **788.30** (Incontinence), **V10.46** (History, personal, malignant neoplasm, prostate)

83. Report 82: **52630** (Transurethral Procedure, Prostate, Resection)

85. Report 84: **53852** (Transurethral Procedure, Prostate, Thermotherapy, Radiofrequency), **76872** (Ultrasound, rectal)

CHAPTER 21: REPRODUCTIVE, INTERSEX SURGERY, FEMALE GENITAL SYSTEM, AND MATERNITY CARE AND DELIVERY

Theory

Female Genital Terminology

1. d

3. h

5. b

7. m

9. c

Copyright © 2016 by Elsevier Inc.

11. j

13. f

Maternity Care and Delivery Terminology

15. e

17. g

19. f

21. j

23. l

25. o

27. i

29. n

31. introitus

33. colpocentesis

35. False

37. colposcope

39. loop electrode excision procedure

41. hysterectomy

43. Radiology

45. Oviduct/Ovary

47. trimesters

49. estimated date (of) delivery

51. E/M

Practical

53. **57400** (Dilation, Vagina)

55. **56441** (Adhesions, Labial, Lysis)

57. **58558** (Hysteroscopy, Surgical with Biopsy)

59. **58920** (Ovary, Wedge Resection)

61. **58800** (Cyst, Ovarian, Incision and Drainage)

63. **59514** (Cesarean Delivery, Delivery Only)

65. **59020** (Fetal Contraction Stress Test)

67. **56440** (Marsupialization, Cyst, Bartholin's Gland)

69. **57065** (Destruction, Lesion, Vagina, Extensive)

Reports

71. Report 28: **59409** (Vaginal Delivery, Delivery Only)

    ICD-10-CM: **O76** (Delivery, complicated by, fetal, heart rate or rhythm), **O66.0** (Delivery, complicated, by, obstruction, due to, dystocia, shoulder), **O70.1** (Delivery, complicated, by, laceration, perineum, second degree), **Z37.0** (Outcome of delivery, single liveborn).

    ICD-9-CM: **669.51** (Delivery, vacuum extractor), **659.71** (Delivery, fetal, heart rate or rhythm), **652.81** (Delivery, complicated, shoulder, presentation), **664.11** (Delivery, complicated, laceration, perineum, second degree, delivered), **V27.0** (Outcome of delivery, single liveborn)

Copyright © 2016 by Elsevier Inc.

Note: You report the delivery only because by reading this note you have no idea if the delivering physician was her regular obstetrician before and after delivery care.

73. Report 30: **59000** (Amniocentesis, Diagnostic)

    ICD-10-CM: **O09.293** (Pregnancy, complicated by, poor obstetric history), **Z36** (Screening [for], antenatal [of mother]), **Z87.448** (History, personal, disease or disorder, urinary system NEC)

    ICD-9-CM: **V23.49** (History of, obstetrical disorder, affecting management of current, pregnancy), **V28.2** (Screening [for] antenatal, of mother, based on amniocentesis), **V13.09** (History, personal, disorder, urinary system, specified NEC)

CHAPTER 22: ENDOCRINE AND NERVOUS SYSTEMS

Theory

Endocrine System Terminology

1. c
3. f
5. d
7. g
9. h
11. b

Nervous System Terminology

13. g
15. h
17. b
19. d

Practical

21. **60000** (Thyroid Gland, Cyst, Incision and Drainage)
23. **64840** (Suture, Nerve)
25. **64831** (Repair, Nerve, Suture), **69990** (Operating Microscope)
27. **62311** (Injection, Spinal Cord, Anesthetic)
29. **61619** (Skull Base Surgery, Dura, Repair of Cerebrospinal Fluid Leak)
31. **63030** (Hemilaminectomy), **63035** (Hemilaminectomy)

Reports

33. Report 43: **63030-RT** (Hemilaminectomy)

    ICD-10-CM: **M51.16** (Displacement, intervertebral disc, lumbar, with neuritis, radiculitis, sciatica, or other pain)

    ICD-9-CM: **722.10** (Displacement, intervertebral disc, [with neuritis, radiculitis, sciatica, or other pain], lumbar)

Copyright © 2016 by Elsevier Inc.

CHAPTER 23: EYE, OCULAR ADNEXA, AUDITORY, AND OPERATING MICROSCOPE

Theory

Eye and Ocular Adnexa Terminology

1. a
3. b
5. c
7. d
9. i
11. g
13. k
15. f
17. d
19. h
21. j

Auditory System Terminology

23. g
25. n
27. h
29. i
31. k
33. a
35. c
37. l

Practical

39. **67570-RT** (Decompression, Optic Nerve)
41. **69620-LT** (Myringoplasty)
43. **69661** (Stapedectomy, with Footplate Drill Out)

Reports

45. Report 85: **66720-RT** (Glaucoma, Cryotherapy)
    ICD-10-CM: **H40.10X3** (Glaucoma, open-angle)
    ICD-9-CM: **365.10** (Glaucoma, open-angle); **365.73** (Glaucoma, severe stage)
47. Report 87: **66984-RT** (Cataract, Removal, Extraction, Extracapsular)

CHAPTER 24: RADIOLOGY

Theory

1. c
3. b
5. a
7. b
9. f

Copyright © 2016 by Elsevier Inc.

11. a

13. e

15. i

17. h

19. j

21. c

Practical

23. **78499** (Unlisted Services and Procedures, Nuclear Medicine, Heart)

25. -26

27. **75705** (Angiography, Spinal Artery)

29. **70130** (X-Ray, Mastoids)

31. **70542** (Magnetic Resonance Imaging [MRI], Diagnostic, Neck)

33. **73502** (X-Ray, Hip)

35. **76098** (X-Ray, Specimen/Surgical)

37. **99219** for initial observation care (Evaluation and Management, Hospital Services, Observation Care); **70450** for CT Scan without mention of contrast (CT Scan, without Contrast), **76516** for A-scan (Ultrasound, Eye, Biometry); **77261** for therapeutic radiation (Radiation Therapy Planning); **77402** simple radiation delivery (Radiation Therapy, Treatment Delivery, Single); **77427** for weekly radiology therapy management (Radiation Therapy, Treatment Management, Weekly)

39. **76604** (Ultrasound, Chest); **71550** for the MRI (Magnetic Resonance Imaging [MRI], Diagnostic, Chest); **33020** for the pericardiotomy (Pericardiotomy, Removal, Clot)

41. **73092** (X-Ray, Arm, Upper)

43. **77002** (Fluoroscopy, Needle Biopsy)

45. **76872** (Ultrasound, Rectal)

47. **72240** (Myelography, Spine, Cervical)

49. **70140** (X-Ray, Facial Bones)

51. **74010** (X-Ray, Abdomen)

53. **75870** (Venography, Sagittal Sinus)

    ICD-10-CM: **G08** (Thrombosis, sinus, intracranial)

    ICD-9-CM: **325** (Thrombosis, sinus, intracranial)

55. **37252** (Ultrasound, Non-Coronary, Intravascular)

    ICD-10-CM: **I70.1** (Stenosis, artery, renal)

    ICD-9-CM: **440.1** (Stenosis, artery, renal)

Reports

57. Report 45: **71010** (X-Ray, Chest)

    ICD-10-CM: **R07.9** (Pain, chest)

    ICD-9-CM: **786.50** (Pain, chest)

59. Report 47: **70480-26** (CT Scan, without Contrast, Orbit)

    ICD-10-CM: **H57.12** (Pain, eye)

    ICD-9-CM: **379.91** (Pain[s], ocular)

Copyright © 2016 by Elsevier Inc.

61. Report 49: **74000-26** (X-Ray, Abdomen)

    ICD-10-CM: **E46** (Malnutrition)

    ICD-9-CM: **263.9** (Malnutrition)

63. Report 51: **74160-26** (CT, with Contrast, Abdomen)

    ICD-10-CM: **R94.5** (Findings, abnormal, inconclusive, function study, liver)

    ICD-9-CM: **794.8** (Findings, abnormal, function study, liver)

65. Report 53: **78451-26** (Myocardial, Perfusion Imaging)

    ICD-10-CM: **R07.9** (Pain[s], chest), **R06.02** (Shortness, breath)

    ICD-9-CM: **786.50** (Pain, chest), **786.05** (Shortness, breath)

CHAPTER 25: PATHOLOGY/LABORATORY

Theory

1. Surgery

3. presence, amount or amount, presence

5. section

7. one

Practical

9. **84520** (Urea Nitrogen, Quantitative), **84295** (Sodium), **84132** (Potassium), **82565** (Creatinine, Blood), **84550** (Uric Acid, Blood)

    ICD-10-CM: **E86.0** (Dehydration), **M25.50** (Pain, joint), **R50.9** (Fever)

    ICD-9-CM: **276.51** (Dehydration), **719.40** (Pain, joint), **780.60** (Fever)

    Note: The Blood Urea Nitrogen (BUN) is part of the blood chemistry for this patient, and there are two codes for blood as the source of the sample—84520 and 84525. Although there are other CPT codes to identify urea nitrogen, the source of the sample for those codes is the urine (84540, 84545).

11. **80076** (Blood Tests, Panels, Hepatic Function), **80061** (Blood Tests, Panels, Lipid Panel)

    ICD-10-CM: **E78.5** (Hyperlipidemia)

    ICD-9-CM: **272.4** (Hyperlipidemia)

13. **80162** (Therapeutic Drug Assay, Digoxin)

    ICD-10-CM: **I48.2** (Fibrillation, atrial or auricular, chronic)

    ICD-9-CM: **427.31** (Fibrillation, atrial)

Reports

15. Report 55: **88305** Urinary Bladder (Pathology, Surgical, Gross and Micro Exam, Level IV)

    ICD-10-CM: **D09.0** (Neoplasm, bladder, Malignant Ca in-situ)

    ICD-9-CM: **233.7** (Neoplasm, bladder, Malignant, Ca in situ)

17. Report 57: **88304** Intervertebral Disc (Pathology, Surgical, Gross and Micro Exam, Level III)

    ICD-10-CM: **M51.26** (Displacement, intervertebral disc, lumbar region)

    ICD-9-CM: **722.10** (Displacement, intervertebral disc, lumbar, lumbosacral)

Copyright © 2016 by Elsevier Inc.

19. Report 59: **88305** Muscle (Pathology, Surgical, Gross and Micro Exam, Level IV)

    ICD-10-CM: **D17.1** (Lipoma, trunk)

    ICD-9-CM: **728.2** (Atrophy, muscle, muscular)

21. Report 61: **88304** Skin Cyst (Pathology, Surgical, Gross and Micro Exam, Level III)

    ICD-10-CM: **L72.9** (Cyst, skin)

    ICD-9-CM: **706.2** (Cyst, skin)

23. Report 63: **88307** Liver (Pathology, Surgical, Gross and Micro Exam, Level V)

    ICD-10-CM: **E66.01** (Obesity, morbid), **K76.0** (Fatty, liver)

    ICD-9-CM: **278.01** (Obesity, morbid); **571.8** (Fatty, liver)

25. Report 65: **88309** Lung Lobe (Pathology, Surgical, Gross and Micro Exam, Level VI)

    ICD-10-CM: **J85.2** (Abscess, lung)

    ICD-9-CM: **513.0** (Abscess, lung)

27. Report 67: **88104** (Cytopathology, Fluids, Washings, Brushings, Smears)

    ICD-10-CM: **J90** (Effusion, pleura)

    ICD-9-CM: **511.9** (Effusion, pleura)

CHAPTER 26: MEDICINE

Theory

1. m
3. h
5. n
7. i
9. g
11. l
13. a
15. g
17. f
19. a
21. c
23. hearing test
25. stimulation of the cochlea to measure electrical activity
27. studying the capillaries of the eyes
29. a device for detecting color blindness
31. cornea and sclera together forming one organ
33. the thick outer coat of the eye, mostly white and opaque

Practical

35. **95052 × 2** (Allergy Tests, Patch, Photo Patch)
37. **92341** (Spectacle Services, Fitting, Spectacles)
39. **92534** (Nystagmus Tests, Optokinetic)
41. **91034** (Esophagus, Acid Reflux Tests)

43. **90880** (Hypnotherapy)

45. **92626** (Rehabilitation, Auditory, Status Evaluation)

47. **90940** (Hemodialysis, Blood Flow Study)

49. **93503** (Cardiac Catheterization, Insertion, Flow Directed Catheter, Swan Ganz)

51. **94003** (Ventilation Assist)

    ICD-10-CM: **J96.00** (Failure, respiration, respiratory, acute)

    ICD-9-CM: **518.81** (Failure, respiration, respiratory, acute)

53. **99144** (Sedation, Moderate)

55. **90471** (Administration, Immunization, One Vaccine/Toxoid), **90472** (Administration, Immunization, each additional Vaccine/Toxoid)

57. ICD-10-CM: **I21.19** (Infarct, myocardium, ST elevation, inferior [inferolateral]), **I23.1** (Defect, atrial septal, following acute myocardial infarction)

    ICD-9-CM: **410.21** (Infarct, myocardium), **429.71** (Defect, atrial septal, acquired)

Reports

59. Report 68: **99203** (Office and/or Other Outpatient Services, New Patient)

    ICD-10-CM: **I25.10** (Arteriosclerosis, coronary), **I10** (Hypertension), **N63** (Mass, breast), **Z95.1** (Status, aortacoronary bypass), **Z79.890** (Long-term, hormone replacement), **Z82.49** (History, family, disease or disorder, cardiovascular disease), **Z80.3** (History, family, malignant neoplasm, breast)

    ICD-9-CM: **414.01** (Arteriosclerosis, coronary, native artery), **401.9** (Hypertension, Unspecified), **611.72** (Mass, breast), **V45.81** (Status, coronary artery bypass), **V49.81** (Status, postmenopausal), **V17.49** (History, family, cardiovascular disease), **V16.3** (History, family, malignant neoplasm, breast)

61. Report 70: **99241** (Consultation, Office and/or Other Outpatient)

63. Report 72: **none**, as the admission is part of the surgical package

65. Report 74: **19307-LT** (Mastectomy, Modified Radical)

    ICD-10-CM: **C50.912** (Neoplasm, breast, Malignant Primary)

    ICD-9-CM: **174.9** (Neoplasm, breast, Malignant, Primary)

67. Report 76: **99252-57** (Consultation, Inpatient) modifier -57 indicates the decision for major surgery

    ICD-10-CM: **I97.89** (Complication, circulatory, system, post procedural), **M79.606** (Pain, limb, lower)

    ICD-9-CM: **997.79** (Complication, vascular, postoperative, other vessels) for postoperative vascular complications, **729.5** (Pain, leg)

69. Report 78: **32554** (Thoracentesis)

    ICD-10-CM: **J90** (Effusion, pleural)

    ICD-9-CM: **511.9** (Effusion, pleura). Note that the report indicated the patient was developing respiratory failure; if the failure was confirmed, the diagnosis would be reported with **518.81** (Respiratory, failure).

    Note: The report indicated the patient was developing respiratory failure; if the failure was confirmed, the diagnosis would be reported with **J96.00** (Failure, respiration, respiratory, acute).

Copyright © 2016 by Elsevier Inc.

71. Report 80: **94060** (Spirometry), **94729** (Pulmonology, Diagnostic, Carbon Monoxide Diffusion Capacity), **99070** (Supplies, Materials) for the bronchodilator

CHAPTER 27: INPATIENT CODING

Theory

1. Inpatient
3. Outpatient
5. False
7. False
9. a
11. b
13. c
15. c

Sequencing Exercises

Cases of Principal Diagnosis and Other Diagnoses

17. Principal diagnosis: congestive heart failure
    Other diagnoses: none
19. Principal diagnosis: postoperative hemorrhage
    Other diagnoses: ovarian cancer, primary
21. Principal diagnosis: third-degree burn to arm/stomach (either the arm or the stomach could be sequenced first)
    Other diagnoses: second-degree burn thigh
23. Principal diagnosis: dehydration
    Other diagnoses: gastroenteritis
    Pregnancy is reported with a V code for incidental state.

Principal Diagnosis

25. **ICD-10-CM: Principal diagnosis and code:** Right posterior and anterior communicating artery aneurysm **I67.1** (Aneurysm, brain)
    Other diagnosis and code: Right otitis externa **H60.391** (Otitis, externa)
    Procedure: 03VG0ZZ Right craniotomy for clipping of arterial aneurysm (Restriction, Artery, Intracranial)
    ICD-9-CM: **Principal diagnosis and code: 437.3** (Aneurysm, brain)
    Other diagnosis and code: 380.10 (Otitis, external)
    Procedure: 39.51 (Clipping, aneurysm)

Copyright © 2016 by Elsevier Inc.

Step 2: Practice

"Before everything else, getting ready is the secret of success."

— Henry Ford

Thank you for pursuing excellence in your coding education!

As coding becomes a more complex and specialized career, it is extremely important that we coders stay at the top of our coding game. That's why, as lifelong coders and educators, we know that tools for more advanced learning and practice are crucial for today's top coders.

Thank you for being committed to being one of the best and rising to the top in your career.

— Carol J. Buck,
MS, CPC, CCS-P

— Jackie L. Grass,
CPC

Track your progress!

See the checklist in the back of this book
to learn more about your next step toward coding success!

Step 3: Certify

Congratulations on reaching the certification step in your career!

As you know, certified coders are in top demand in today's marketplace. That's why, as lifelong coders and educators, we have dedicated ourselves to providing the most up-to-date, comprehensive, and user-friendly certification review books on the market. We update these books every year so that you will have the best tools possible when studying for your certification exam. It's time to hit the books.

You can do it! We know you can!

— Carol J. Buck,
MS, CPC, CCS-P

— Jackie L. Grass,
CPC

Track your progress!

See the checklist in the back of this book
to learn more about your next step toward coding success!

BB-03

Step 4:
Professional Resources

"Nothing is particularly hard if you divide it into small jobs."

— Henry Ford

As you reach higher and more specialized levels of coding, we want to applaud you for taking this step in your career. You won't be disappointed. Specialized coders are like rare gems—***they are harder to find and greatly valued*** in the profession.

— Carol J. Buck,
MS, CPC, CCS-P

— Jackie L. Grass,
CPC

Track your progress!

**See the checklist in the back of this book
to learn more about your steps toward coding success!**

Sharpen your coding skills

with *interactive study* and *practice* from
Carol J. Buck!

Medical Coding Online
for Step-by-Step Medical
Coding, 2016 Edition

Carol J. Buck, MS, CPC, CCS-P

December 2015 • **ISBN: 978-0-323-38922-8**

This complete online course complements
essential content from your *Step-by-Step*
textbook with practice activities and self-
assessment opportunities to reinforce your
knowledge of essential coding concepts and
help you learn more effectively!

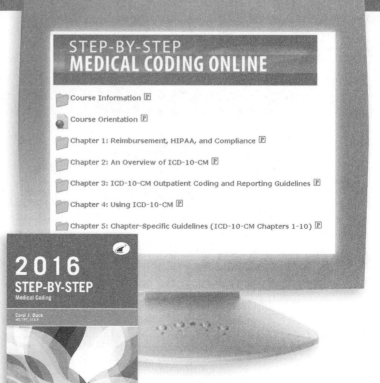

Strengthen your understanding and coding skills with:

- **Interactive coding exercises** that provide valuable, case-based
  practice and challenge you to apply your coding knowledge.

- **Narrated animations** that enhance your understanding of complex concepts
  with engaging visual demonstrations accompanied by expert commentary.

- **Chapter assessment questions** that cover key chapter content
  and help you identify your strengths and weaknesses.

Order today!

- Order securely at **www.elsevier.com.**
- Call toll-free **1-800-545-2522.**
- Visit your **local bookstore.**

ELSEVIER

MCO-01

Trust Carol J. Buck
for your certification review needs!

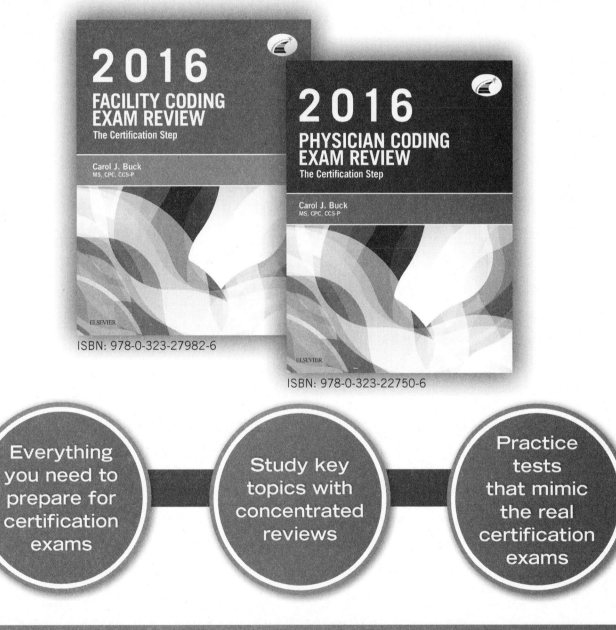

2016 FACILITY CODING EXAM REVIEW
The Certification Step
Carol J. Buck
MS, CPC, CCS-P
ELSEVIER
ISBN: 978-0-323-27982-6

2016 PHYSICIAN CODING EXAM REVIEW
The Certification Step
Carol J. Buck
MS, CPC, CCS-P
ELSEVIER
ISBN: 978-0-323-22750-6

Everything you need to prepare for certification exams

Study key topics with concentrated reviews

Practice tests that mimic the real certification exams

Order today!
- Order securely at **www.elsevier.com.**
- Call toll-free **1-800-545-2522.**
- Visit your **local bookstore.**

ELSEVIER

CERT-01